Action Research in Health Care

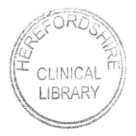

Other books of interest:

D.F.S. Cormack
The Research Process in Nursing
Fourth Edition
0-632-05158-2

I. Holloway & S. Wheeler
Qualitative Research for Nurses
0-632-03765-2

I. Holloway & S. Walker
Getting a PhD in Health and Social Care
0-632-05057-8

I. Holloway
Basic Concepts for Qualitative Research
0-632-04173-0

Action Research in Health Care

ALISON MORTON-COOPER
PhD, MEd, RN
Researcher-Practitioner in Continuing Education
and Associate Fellow
Department of Continuing Education
University of Warwick

**Blackwell
Science**

Copyright © Alison Morton-Cooper 2000
Blackwell Science Ltd
Editorial Offices:
Osney Mead, Oxford OX2 0EL
25 John Street, London WC1N 2BL
23 Ainslie Place, Edinburgh EH3 6AJ
350 Main Street, Malden
   MA 02148 5018, USA
54 University Street, Carlton
   Victoria 3053, Australia
10, rue Casimir Delavigne
   75006 Paris, France

Other Editorial Offices:

Blackwell Wissenschafts-Verlag GmbH
Kurfürstendamm 57
10707 Berlin, Germany

Blackwell Science KK
MG Kodenmacho Building
7–10 Kodenmacho Nihombashi
Chuo-ku, Tokyo 104, Japan

First published 2000

Set in 10.5/14 Meridien
by Sparks Computer Solutions Ltd, Oxford
Printed and bound in Great Britain by
MPG Books Ltd, Bodmin, Cornwall

The Blackwell Science logo is a
trade mark of Blackwell Science Ltd,
registered at the United Kingdom
Trade Marks Registry

DISTRIBUTORS

Marston Book Services Ltd
PO Box 269
Abingdon
Oxon OX14 4YN
(*Orders:* Tel: 01235 465500
         Fax: 01235 465555)

USA
Blackwell Science, Inc.
Commerce Place
350 Main Street
Malden, MA 02148 5018
(*Orders:* Tel: 800 759 6102
           781 388 8250
         Fax: 781 388 8255)

Canada
Login Brothers Book Company
324 Saulteaux Crescent
Winnipeg, Manitoba R3J 3T2
(*Orders:* Tel: 204 837-2987
         Fax: 204 837-3116)

Australia
Blackwell Science Pty Ltd
54 University Street
Carlton, Victoria 3053
(*Orders:* Tel: 03 9347 0300
         Fax: 03 9347 5001)

A catalogue record for this title
is available from the British Library

ISBN 0-632-04091-2

Library of Congress
Cataloging-in-Publication Data
Morton-Cooper, Alison
  Action research in health care / Alison-
    Morton-Cooper.
    p. cm
  Includes bibliographical references and index
  ISBN 0-632-04091-2
  1. Action research. 2. Medical care—
    Research—Methodology. I. Title.

RA440.85 .M67 2000
362.1'07'2—dc21   99-087086

For further information on
Blackwell Science, visit our website:
www.blackwell-science.com

Contents

Acknowledgements

Sincere thanks are due to all colleagues, friends and family who continue to share my enthusiasm for action research and to all those who have generously given their unconditional support to my efforts to improve practice over the last twenty years. I am especially indebted to Dr Margaret Bamford for her encouragement and for sharing with me her political acumen and understanding of the ways of the world.

As ever I thank the staff of the libraries of the University of Warwick and the Royal College of Nursing for their help and expertise, and Griselda Campbell and the editorial staff of Blackwell Science for their strategic support and guidance.

Introduction

This book is written in response to all those of you who have struggled in vain to find a practical, concise and yet insightful account of the use of action research methods in health care practice.

The demand for evidence-based, ethically sensitive and clinically effective methods of problem-solving that can help organisations and individuals to focus more clearly on the problems they encounter, and take affirmative action to find workable solutions, increases daily. This is partly in response to government policy initiatives for greater economic and professional accountability, but is also a result of the information overload which has overwhelmed decision-makers and policy-drivers in recent years.

Problems of practice require systematic and rigorous examination, but not all can be made sense of through the conventional methods of positivist scientific scrutiny. The need to develop active rather than passive research tools which involve practitioners and clients in a positive and ethical process of consciousness raising, is becoming greater as we try to make collective and personal sense of the many changes in our midst.

Active research methods which help practitioners to sustain efforts to improve and change practice for the better, while at the same time acknowledging and respecting the contribution of individuals to the change process, offer a glimmer of hope to those who have found themselves frustrated by traditional research methods based on quantitative analysis and control.

Living and working in the messy, constantly evolving health care scenario requires more innovative and flexible methods of exploration than have hitherto been made possible under the canon of medical scientific method, the so-called 'gold standard' of research into health.

Health *care*, I would argue, needs a more person-sensitive approach; practitioners deal in the end not with the masses, but with individuals and their families, a fact which most medical model research studies fail to take into account. The care we provide, and the quality of the professional relationship we enter into, is very much based on the here and now and not on the hypothetical situation so typical of psychologically distanced studies. The latter approach seeks to address disease as a process rather than to make a human response to health problems and their real-life consequences.

Action research has grown in stature in the fields of education and industry because it centres on people and their problems. Thus it necessarily shares aspects of their human frailty and apparent fickleness: it refuses to be bound by the conventional methods used to create boundaries in scientific research. Rather, it has a tendency to reflect and become caught up in the hubbub of human activity 'out there' in the research environment, and presents particular challenges to the research community and to practitioners. In these days of clinical governance it provides a valuable means of developing responsible and reflective practice which takes into account the different stakeholders within a public service environment.

Action research is a cyclical process which begins by asking a group of people to examine a problem within their culture and to find ways of solving or reducing that problem. Each person involved, including the researcher who initiates the process, becomes part of the action research network and *involves themselves fully* in articulating the problem and envisioning possible solutions. This is very much a hands-on method of researching social life, with everyone involved becoming an actor in the encounters described.

Perhaps this is why the professions close to medicine are beginning to recognise its worth. Few other approaches are so effective in rooting out the source of problems in practice and in challenging the status quo. As part of the action research process it is possible to discover things about ourselves which were previously unknown or unacknowledged. The insights derived from action research are not always comfortable or those we would like to see, rather they require an ability to be brave and to confront problems which we may have previously neglected. Action research is a political activity, based on ideas about social justice and democratic forms of participation in the research process.

This can test our beliefs about our relationships and ways of working and may require a reappraisal of how we came to be where we are and the directions in which we are headed as we encounter the future. Experienced action researchers will tell you that their involvement with action research changed their lives and their way of looking at the world. By uncovering the chaos surrounding them, paradoxically, they were able to identify islands of thought which, when brought together, helped them to clarify and address their problems anew.

There are excellent texts on the market which can help readers to get to grips more fully with the history and philosophy of action research and these will be signposted as appropriate. This book seeks to:

- explain the ethos and principles of action research;
- demonstrate how it may be used in health care practice;
- help practitioners participate in and/or plan, carry out and evaluate their own action research studies in ways which are appropriate for them personally and professionally;
- assist students undertaking research degrees or projects based on action research to manage the action research process with confidence and conviction; and
- provide insight into action research for professionals in health care and academia which can help them to support employees or students involved in action research.

Contents of the book

The book is divided into four chapters, the first of which outlines the *principles of action research design*, together with a brief discussion about the history, aims and ethos of the method. The characteristics of an effective action researcher are mooted, to give some flavour of what it means to become involved in a study of this kind.

A further discussion on the various applications of action research (AR) methodology is included at this early stage to illustrate why some action researchers come unstuck early in the process, largely because the approach taken was inappropriate to their particular research question.

This chapter ends with the question 'Why choose action research?' so that those of you who have been contemplating an AR study will be able to articulate a clear justification for its use.

Chapter 2 discusses prioritising and the various processes involved in *preparing a research proposal* and obtaining logistic and financial support for your work. Issues include planning, research ethics, collaborative literature reviewing, and choosing a setting for your study. Practitioners who are research students are also offered some advice here. The collaborative nature of action research requires careful planning and effective communication strategies. By the end of this chapter you should feel confident about the resources needed to get your study off the ground, and have a realistic idea of how you are going to manage these.

The third chapter is essentially about *managing your fieldwork*, beginning with the clarification of aims and values inherent in the study and followed up by a detailed consideration of how you intend to manage your study, the relationships which emerge from your involvement, the process of data collection and the management of information and feedback processes over time. Researcher professionalism is a vital prerequisite to gaining credibility in the field and in helping to see that your work constitutes a valid account of what is happening. Data collection is an enormously challenging stage in research work, particularly when your study is highly qualitative. There are some very effective strategies available to help you deal with the feeling of rising panic which can ensue when the data 'mountain' threatens to overwhelm you, so read this chapter carefully, particularly if this is your first foray into research territory.

Analysis and interpretation are the touchstones of qualitative research. This stage of the research has the potential to be very rewarding intellectually and socially, and Chapter 4 is intended to help you make the best of this stage. Staying motivated has much to do with your collective and personal ability to 'grow' with the data, and this chapter has a particular concern with helping you to manage the change which accompanies action research in as constructive a way as possible.

Writing up your analysis and findings is the part which many people put off for longest. Chapter 4 explores the issues and practicalities involved and offers tips for surviving what is undoubtedly a most politically sensitive part of the action research process. The next critical step of publishing and disseminating your work is highlighted and some suggestions made as to how you can manage this process.

Critical review is an essential part of keeping our work alive and meaningful and an Appendix contains guidelines for critiquing both your own work and published studies based on action research. References for all chapters are placed at the end of the book, together with suggestions for further reading aimed mainly at beginning researchers and practitioners becoming involved in an action research study for the first time.

Action research in health care is something of a 'new age' approach, and it is only beginning to be recognised and acknowledged for its tremendous potential in bringing professionals and their patients and clients closer together. No writer can hope to provide the definitive guide to action research in health care as it is too young a philosophy to have gained enough ground. I do hope that what you read – which is really only the sum of my own fairly extensive engagement with action research communities – provides some encouragement and insight into what will I know be an exciting, intellectually stimulating and formative experience in any health professional's career.

Whether you are an experienced advocate of action research or someone who has an interest in finding out more, I wish you well. Together, we *can* and *will* change the world!

Alison Morton-Cooper
Castle Douglas, 1999

CHAPTER 1

Principles of action research design

Action research as a dynamic alternative to traditional scientific method

For natural scientists who seek to explain and predict nature, science itself is a calm, rational and justifiable response to the problems which threaten our very existence. In order to manipulate our environment and survive, we look to science for the answers it can provide to very urgent and important questions. Without the ability to observe, quantify, describe and predict, we would not have been able even to try to solve the critical threats posed by disease and famine, to wonder at the ways in which disease can be prevented, and to marvel at the pharmacological solutions to intransigent problems which can spread remorselessly without human intervention.

As our knowledge of, for example, human genetics increases so does our potential to predict the future. Anything, it is now clear, may be possible: science in the twenty-first century will produce new species, diagnose illness long before symptoms appear, 'know' human beings at the biochemical level, manipulate reproduction and change ourselves (Appleyard 1999: 15, 23, 26).

Given the colossal claims for science, it is easy to see why some scientists become so engrossed in their quest for progress that their vision fails to take account of the individual nature of what it means to be a passive recipient of its wisdom.

Medical science in particular seeks to distance itself from the fleshy reality of humankind. Its purpose lies in setting deterministic models which predict future events, all the better for clinicians to base clinical decisions on probabilities (Alasuutari 1998).

The ability to reflect on evidence, and more important to reflect critically, has become an essential skill for the clinician of the future (Pietroni 1998). The problem remains, however, that methods which seek to explain and predict at some distance from the ultimate recipients are not especially successful at helping practitioners and carers to deliver care appropriately, given the individual patient's need for understanding and an appreciation of their personal situation. Conventional health research can help to illuminate trends within populations and the physical processes involved in the progress of a disease; what it cannot do is help us to apply our new-found knowledge with any more sensitivity, skill or expertise than before.

We have all met practitioners who are extremely well-informed about their specialisms in terms of factual knowledge, but who fail to understand the requirements of patients and clients who do not engage in the scientific discourse *clinical* thinking brings about.

Sociologists have built careers around the ways in which patients and practitioners interact and 'live' in the clinical domain, with patients being viewed as the passive and relatively powerless consumers of knowledge passed down to them from on high and, ultimately, as a cultural product of 'scientific progress'.

The intention here is not to disparage positivist enquiry, or to underestimate its power for good. Rather, it is to establish a backdrop for the consideration of what will instead be described as *un*conventional science, the so-called 'new paradigm' research partly constituted by action research in health care practice.

Passion, for example, is not something we normally associate with good research, largely, it could be supposed, because of its emotiveness, the sense in which it is thought to constitute a departure from our ideas of control. Conventionally, therefore, a scientist must be wary of, and take care to avoid, passion, lest he or she be carried along by its irrationality and forget the need for cool, considered objectivity in the face of the evidence.

On the contrary, in order to succeed, action researchers need to engage actively and with passion in the research process. Passive, dispassionate involvement is considered sterile in action research. Without active engagement and personal as well as collective commitment to its aims, action research withers and dies on the vine. Action research has failed if it has not succeeded in bringing to life the people and the purpose for which the research is designed. Action research describes a real-world intervention in a real-life scenario and in many ways it is dramatic, contentious and fraught with inconsistency and unpredictability.

In theory then, action research appears to be at odds with the values and philosophical tenets of ostensibly objective and historically dominant methodological approaches. However, the two positions are closer philosophically than some might think, having the common goal of advancing and adding to the body of knowledge and ideas on a given subject. An important caveat is that action research begins with the stated intention of *improving practice* as well as producing additional knowledge. Action research is in some ways a celebration of human subjectivity, which harnesses a variety of different techniques to qualitatively interpret progress made through the process of research, rather than seeking to quantify and measure its effects by traditional laboratory-influenced methods.

It therefore makes no claims to be value-free as conventional scientific research requires, rather it acknowledges the value-laden nature of human research activity, and attempts to communicate the human contribution to progress in a way which would not be acceptable to arch-positivists.

To see how we arrived at such a position let us examine what researchers mean by an action research stance.

What is action research?

In order to get some grasp of how action research has evolved into the different conceptualisations it now enjoys in different areas of professional practice, we need first of all to look at its early history and development.

The early history of action research has been traced to the work of social psychologist Kurt Lewin at the Center for Group Dynamics, Massachusetts Institute of Technology in Boston, USA, in the 1940s, and to a group of war-time researchers in London, from which evolved the Tavistock Institute of Human Relations. Both groups were interested in working collaboratively with employees and their managers in order to understand and study the problems affecting them (Barton-Cunningham 1993).

As social research methods developed, interest in the idea of feedback techniques which monitored attitudes and feelings about work problems grew, fuelled by the growing recognition that workers interact with their work environment and are not simply passive doers or bystanders in the workplace (*ibid.* 16).

This was in stark contrast to other prevailing post-war theories about people and organisations, which had come about in response to different cultural perspectives on management, influenced by the work of F.W. Taylor in the US (scientific management), Henri Fayol in France (the 'administrative model') and Max Weber's ideas about bureaucracy in Germany (Schneider & Barsoux 1997).

The Taylorist idea that workers were driven mainly by economic reward and were best controlled through authority was viewed positively by governments of the time, and was largely accepted as the 'rational' response to the post-war economic drive for stability. Work practices in the post-war years were thus characterised by centralised control of work processes and lack of worker autonomy (Stead & Lee 1996).

Worker identity metamorphosed into a mass, relatively homogenous, semi-skilled workforce involved in large-scale production activities and supported by bureaucratic systems of management. Compared to today's fragmented and 'flexible' workforce, these workers enjoyed (or endured?) stable, long-term organisational careers, typified by production workers constructing Ford motor cars in factory settings, hence the term Fordism used in the literature by economists, labour theorists and, more recently, human resource developers (see Crompton *et al.* 1996).

Steadfastly rejecting the view that people were only cogs to be oiled in the manufacturing machine, social scientists influenced by democratic values and concern with the costs of such autocratic management began studying the notion of worker participation in decision-making. It was not until the 1970s and studies on the quality of work life (QWL) that researchers began to pay sustained attention to the possibilities for increasing efficiency by encouraging worker participation (Whyte 1991).

Kurt Lewin had developed his own interest in the psychological study of human issues after taking up an academic career in the US, having sought refuge from Nazi Germany in 1933. He had grown particularly concerned with the difficulties faced by minority groups and, according to Barton-Cunningham, wanted to build a 'bridge between social theory and social action' by helping individuals to establish their place *within the group* as a source of social status and fundamental, existential security (Barton-Cunningham 1993: 12).

Lewin's approach is described as set apart from other social research in two ways, firstly by studying a given society or community in *motion*, as it were, and in its distinctive view that the nature and meaning of social scientific knowledge, and thus its purpose, lies in its ability to change social reality (Alasuutari 1998: 89). Lewin saw group situations (and thus organisations) as malleable and dynamic, rather than static and predictable. This constituted a significant and far-sighted advance on contemporary orthodox psychologists who subscribed to the view that all human behaviour was driven by immutable laws and could therefore be studied and manipulated by employers to best effect (a view still adhered to by proponents of psychometric testing today).

Communities of workers were no longer to be seen as low-ranking and therefore excluded from potential decision-making, but as influential participants in a social process, much of which was therefore open to critical analysis and interpretation.

Lewin's ideas about human and personal development have since pervaded a good deal of thinking in industrial psychology and management theory, but have probably been interpreted most literally by educationalists who have adopted the ethos of action research into education literature by viewing it as a means for improving education practice and teacher development, particularly in mainstream education (see, for example, Winter 1989, Elliott 1991).

Action research appears to have branched into several directions at this point: as a form of operations and group dynamics research in industry; as a means of engaging in psychoanalytic person-centred research in human relations theory; and as a form of personal and professional development and a means of improving professional practice in the respective fields of education, health and social welfare.

The ethos of action research is perhaps best expressed in the work of Jean McNiff and her colleagues when they write about the process of 'creating a good social order through action research' (McNiff et al. 1992). This echoes the sentiment of Lewin's work which, far from seeing predictable laws inherent in social life, views people as dynamic agents in their own destinies, capable of making a difference to the world by collective and concerted action. In arriving at a rationale for action research, therefore, 'the *social* basis of action research is *involvement*; the *educational* basis is *improvement*...' (McNiff 1988: 3, my italics).

If we want to define action research, then, we need to study its evolution from our own professional perspectives.

Stringer, for example, has interpreted it as a community-based model of research practice with a very clearly defined emphasis on social action. In his view, community-based action research *'is a collaborative approach to inquiry or investigation that provides people with the means to take systematic action to resolve specific problems'*. In Stringer's words this approach favours consensual and participatory procedures that enable people to systematically investigate problems and issues for themselves; to formulate powerful and sophisticated accounts of their situations, and finally, to devise plans to deal with the problem at hand (Stringer 1996: 15).

Thus community-based action research strategies have been used to investigate issues of concern to social planners. A good example is the work of Doyle and colleagues who studied issues of access and equity to social and health services for ethnic groups across a city population in Canada. This approach helped researchers to identify key weaknesses in securing access to services and demonstrated felt concern regarding the attitudes and approachability of staff who were in a position to help people. The 'program for action' which followed addressed the move for change in various areas, such as community outreach, staff recruitment, personnel administration, communications, policy development and training and education strategies amongst others (Doyle 1996: 55).

As an educationalist, Winter takes a different stance, conceptualising action research *'as a way of investigating professional experience which links practice and the analysis of practice into a single, continuously developing sequence'* (Winter 1996: 13). From this perspective, action research 'improves practice by developing the practitioner's capacity for discrimination and judgement in particular, complex, human situations. It unifies inquiry, the improvement of performance and the development of persons in their professional role' (Elliott 1991: 52).

This description is therefore a crystallised interpretation of Lewin's ideas, marked out by the attention it pays to uncovering the norms and values of what constitutes a professional role in society. Action research can help teachers to observe, describe and discuss what is going on in a classroom, for example, and to work collaboratively with pupils and colleagues to find out how group dynamics operate in a given situation. Thus any differences in perception experienced by participants can be aired, and alternative and perhaps competing explanations explored as a way of increasing mutual understanding.

Action research and health care

For practitioners in health care, action research appears to have evolved more slowly, in response to perceptions of an increasing gap between the aims of practice and the theories used to advocate and support them. Disillusioned with the failed promise of the natural scientific view to provide sufficiently holistic answers, some practitioners have sought alternative and more reflexive methods for studying and changing practice which revolve around localised human problems, rather than the more abstract conceptualisations offered by the biomedical model of research.

This in turn can be traced to more general trends affecting populations as social conditions change and require a more flexible response. As Schratz and Walker (1995) have observed, increasingly, more and more of us depend for our survival on working with cultural knowledge in fast-changing circumstances. The politicisation of research has been accelerated by demographic, workplace and employment changes marked by what they describe as a growing separation of the management of professional work from the work itself, creating a need for better information about the delivery of services and thus the emergence of a discourse about what care delivery and service means (Schratz & Walker 1995: 11). In health care, then, the over-arching aim of action research has been to improve professional practice and raise standards of service provision (Nichols *et al.* 1997).

Action research as social action

Action research can be used to help practitioners critically reflect on and examine their work practices and social interactions, and arrive at some consensus of what kind of services should be provided and why they need to be provided in a particular way. It could therefore be described as a *critically reflexive* model of research, being both practice-based and patient-centred in its philosophical approach.

It could also be argued that action research is not really a research method or even a group of methods at all (although it is often described as such); rather it is a philosophical approach to the study of human problems which helps groups to share and refine their understanding of their situations in a mutually supportive environment.

Critically reflexive forms of action research are a way of creating 'a real-world workshop' (Weil 1997) where claims about what constitutes 'valid' knowledge within a given domain can be critically examined and contested by practitioners themselves, generating new ideas and new ways of thinking, seeing and acting (Weil 1998).

Action research represents a powerful challenge to the status quo, in its scrutiny of entrenched, culture-bound structures, practices and opinions; both at the level of governmental control, and in its evaluation of the work of agencies which contribute to or serve the interests and policies of government. To challenge prevailing scientific (or political) opinion – or dogma, depending on your point of view – is a dangerous occupation for the novice researcher, for they may sail unwittingly into very strong tides.

Action research and its potential to unleash erstwhile quieted opinion is one reason why employers and academia have traditionally been wary of its motives. It is also a significant cause of the queasiness sometimes felt by action researchers who find themselves discouraged by those who oppose it either on political grounds, or because they misunderstand the thinking behind its democratic intent.

Weil points out that traditional positivist research is based on the modernist idea that a 'stable state' is possible (see Schon 1971, Weil 1998). Postmodernist thinkers, however, paint a picture of rising instability and social disorder facing the world, as it realigns modernist thinking with the cultural and economic impact of new, ground-breaking technologies which challenge old boundaries and the sovereignty of nation states to govern independently.

Recent developments and global trends have caused us to question old certainties about social and political life, so that early social theories which sought to explain and predict human behaviour have proved inadequate to the task in the late twentieth century (Smart 1996).

The sociologist, Turner, has argued that this has led us into a paradoxical situation for health, in that the attendant deregulation of economies and services which have emerged as a consequence have a tendency to lead to increased state control and intervention. Thus we may now be moving into a new type of society, which Beck has described as a 'risk society' (Beck 1992).

Also a sociologist, Beck has observed that in traditional and early modern society 'health risks were essentially personal, overt, obvious, observable and palpable' (see Turner 1995: 220). By contrast, in advanced western societies our well-being and security is becoming increasingly dependent on the agencies of the state, such as the police, welfare agencies, hospitals and primary health services.

Clearly, living in an earlier, unmedicalised age, going untreated and caring for one's own family on the basis of limited resources, was risky and could lead to an untimely death. Beck believes that in advanced societies risks are instead *hidden* in our institutions and are not palpable, obvious or observable, except when they are brought to our attention by those who question current practices.

Examples of this might be the scandals of physical and psychological abuse of children in state-funded residential care; neglect of the elderly in care homes; the risks associated with advanced technological procedures; and biochemical threats to safety through the use of questionable pharmaceutical substances and purely profit-led agricultural practices. The history of farming and agricultural practice alone is a clear example of the ways in which dependence on the state, adherence to free market principles and demands for increasing product yields can create many dangers which would have been unthinkable at the beginning of the twentieth century.

The changes which have been brought about in society through the global economy have also created a hierarchy for health, with those at the wealthier (top) end having more chance of good health than those who are poor (see Turner 1995: 221). Even this is not straightforward, however, as in the developed world it is not the level of wealth which is thought to create a healthy society, but the quality of social relationships that provide the best indicators for health (Wilkinson 1996).

Thus it can be argued that, although advanced societies can become wealthier in economic terms, the growth of dependence creating and controlling health agencies risks the further erosion of traditional community values and increasing psychosocial *instability*, a position some would argue is evident in the clear correlation between illness and lack of social support that has been alluded to elsewhere (Radley 1994, Cohen & Wills 1985, Berkman 1984).

Responding to the needs of the *un*stable state and instability in social life therefore requires reflexive, courageous and creative thinking, which is not constrained by outdated and false ideas about the nature of the social order. We should try to devolve rather than 'manage' social and moral development by engaging people in making decisions about their future based on an informed and inclusive position (see Weil 1998).

Critically reflexive action research is therefore based on action, and on participative, collaborative forms of data collection which can be used to change our ways of working and seeing the world. It is not only about developing our own praxis (practice) but about critiquing and changing the world (Jennings 1995).

For practitioners in health care, this may require a certain culture shift, a need to challenge some of the cherished beliefs and established canons of health care research, by grounding theories of health in real-world health care practice.

As Rolfe has so astutely observed, research findings of all kinds might, superficially, appear to be the result of an objective process, 'but that objectivity vanishes as soon as a theorist or practitioner attempts to apply them in the real world' (Rolfe 1996: 1319). He argues that nurses, for example, by adopting the restrictive paradigm of the social sciences, have overlooked what should be research's main function, which is to improve nursing practice by the generation and refining of nursing interventions (Rolfe 1996: 1315). Large-scale, statistically generalisable studies which both the gate-keepers of the nursing profession and the Department of Health favour may be adequate for the construction and testing of theory, he writes, but they tell us nothing about the individualised nursing care which is central to effective nursing practice (Rolfe 1998a: 678).

Practitioners of all therapies who seek out evidence on which to base their practical judgements therefore need to call on research methodologies which help them to understand the privileged relationships they enjoy with their patients as well as the scientific basis for treatments and prescribed therapies. We need to understand the moral and ethical basis for our actions as well as the pragmatic reasons for our interventions. Research which succeeds in reducing the distance between what is practised and what is researched has the potential to motivate practitioners, and to help them integrate research into care as is expected of professional practitioners (Wallis 1998). Caring is, after all, a moral enterprise (Lantos 1997).

Sometimes portrayed as a soft option in conducting social research, then, action research is quite simply the opposite. It requires sound ethical groundwork and a great deal of personal commitment to see it through to its political end. Issues around the politics of action research are many and varied and will be discussed as appropriate in later chapters. For the moment, however, you may be anxious to get on and concentrate on the practicalities of action research, and we can begin here by articulating a working definition of the action research concept.

Defining action research in health care

For most practitioners who generate studies on their own behalf, action research involves a small-scale intervention in a setting, process or treatment, and an evaluation or review of the impact of this process (Holloway & Wheeler 1996). Policies and interventions in care thus become legitimate subjects for study in the workplace or care setting.

Larger scale studies may involve practitioners at several levels of the health hierarchy, and some of the most effective have involved a truly interprofessional approach. In arriving at a working definition of action research in health care then, we could usefully describe it as 'a collaborative intervention in a real-world health care situation to define a problem and explore a possible solution'.

Readers who are experienced in action research will no doubt have their own preferred definition. The various definitions already offered clearly share the same ethos, even though they have a subtly different emphasis. What is vital is that before a group of people enter into a study, each shares and acknowledges a single definition based on mutual values and understanding.

Key principles of action research

Action research as the present author understands and uses it is, in principle:

- practitioner-generated;
- workplace oriented;
- seeks to improve practice;
- starts with a problem shared and experienced by colleagues and/or patients;
- examines key assumptions held by researchers and challenges their validity;
- adopts a flexible trial and error approach;
- accepts that there are no final answers; and
- aims to validate any claims it makes by rigorous justification processes.

These key principles have been adapted from the educational model proposed by McNiff and her colleagues, (see McNiff *et al.* 1992: 3) and have proved enormously resilient, both in theory and for their practical utility.

Action research is therefore *problem-sensing* and *problem-focused*, with the researcher being involved in an immediate and direct way with the problem situation; the aim being to realise a state where the 'ideal' becomes 'real' (Hart & Bond 1995: 52). Rolfe sees it as a way of integrating practice with research in a single act, in preference to the 'top down' hierarchical model of research usually experienced and promoted in the workplace (Rolfe 1998b).

Holter and Schwarz-Barcott see the researcher's role as one which facilitates discussion between practitioners concerning possible conflicts generated by different understandings of a problem, at the level of the individual and/or organisational culture. The emphasis therefore is 'on bringing to the surface the underlying value system, including norms and conflicts which may be at the core of problems identified' (Holter & Schwartz-Barcott 1993: 302).

Action researchers can employ all the usual methods of qualitative enquiry, such as surveys, interviews, documentary and policy analysis, participant observation, focus groups, case studies and nominal group techniques, to name a few. All that is different is that, rather than requiring and negotiating access as an outsider to the setting in which the research is to take place, action researchers participate fully in all the activities, sharing them out and feeding back on progress to their co-researchers in the workplace to a timescale discussed, planned and agreed in advance.

This can be managed in discrete stages which are set out in Box 1.1.

Characteristics of an effective action researcher

The types and contexts of research vary widely and there is no simple way of ensuring that projects will be successful. Four factors are thought to increase the chances that a study will go well, however, and they relate to the researcher personally. They are motivation, emotional support, style and personal qualities (Easterby-Smith *et al.* 1991: 11).

The first three will be considered in more detail in Chapter 2 when we look at putting together a research proposal. The personal qualities needed by researchers, however, are rarely focused on in the research literature, with many qualities being taken for granted. The list of essential characteristics (p. 22) is drawn from the subjective personal experience of the present author, added to information and insight gained from years of reading and co-researching with other practitioners.

Action research makes demands on individuals and groups which other philosophical approaches do not, and it is important

Box 1.1 Stages in the action research process

(1) The individual or group proposing to set up a study meets with interested parties to discuss and clarify the problem to be studied, assisted by an initial review of the relevant literature.

(2) A pilot study may be set up to help establish the position(s) and responsibilities of those involved.

(3) A potential solution or intervention is proposed, discussed and modified.

(4) Ethical issues are considered and permission sought from the relevant agencies and committees.

(5) Documentation is devised to accurately record both the process of data collection and the 'evidence' collected.

(6) The process is planned, communicated and carried out to agreed protocols.

(7) A collaborative analysis of the data and evaluation of the outcomes takes place, drawing on the relevant literature.

(8) Key outcomes are discussed and a report written which communicates these clearly to relevant audiences and stakeholders. Policy changes may be formalised at this stage.

(9) The dissemination and publication stage follows, and for those undertaking a dissertation or project, this is presented as a dissertation or thesis depending on the degree being sought.

(10) A decision is taken as to whether a further intervention is to be attempted, as part of a continuous cycle of reflexive practitioner research.

for novice researchers to appreciate the likely responses required of them.

Essential characteristics

- Stamina (psychological and physical);
- patience;
- determination to succeed;
- the ability to motivate and encourage others;
- analytical skills (these may be rusty to begin with, but will soon sharpen up);
- an abiding interest and curiosity in the subject being studied;
- personal integrity and sensitivity to the positions of others;
- ability to communicate well, both orally and in writing;
- a thick skin ('if you can keep your head when all about you are losing theirs', etc.);
- serenity to accept the things that cannot be changed;
- courage to change the things that can; and
- a professional attitude, i.e. the ability to keep things in perspective and to recognise personal and professional limitations.

There are a few personal qualities which can seriously hamper individuals taking part in action research, and these should be remembered whenever a motivation problem is encountered. Lack of motivation can sometimes be traced back to an individual's particular style of working or personal philosophy, and it is important to recognise and respect these as part of an inclusive research process. People who are very precise in their thinking, and who like to see clear boundaries between research activity and practice, will soon feel insecure within an action research project, as action research is a muddy, murky, messy business reflecting the confusion and lack of coherence to be found in real-world settings.

There is a need to be sensitive to the group dynamics operating within the research community. Research of any kind about practice or social interactions raises issues about the nature of the relationship between the researcher and those being researched. There is a danger of damaging the continuation of research projects if practice issues are dealt with insensitively or exploitatively (Marrow 1998).

Any project will by chance involve practitioners who may not share the same opinions or values. Some people will make this clear from the beginning and may even go so far as to exclude themselves from participation. Others may be reluctant to share their misgivings and present a different kind of problem, by half-hearted participation, for example, or (rarely) by actively working against a group and thereby disabling it by more subtle means.

Awareness of different motivations and organisational pressures can help those initiating the study to identify potential problems ahead of time. It is important, however, to be suitably enabling in your own approach to your colleagues, as they will quickly spot and be resentful of any attempt to impose your will on them, and will take particular offence if there is any suggestion that they are to be patronised or talked down to in any way.

Be prepared to take people of all persuasions on board: it is the only way to ensure that the account you produce at the end of your project is culturally valid and valued. Action research is all about exploring and challenging the diversity of opinion on your subject, and is an extremely effective way of helping groups to clarify their values as a helpful precursor to change (Nolan & Grant 1993).

In summary, then, some flexibility and openness to others' points of view are important prerequisites for any action researcher, and can help to ensure that the results of your study are an accurate reflection of the debates it generates in practice.

One practitioner who survived the process is Kevin Hope, a lecturer in nursing at the University of Manchester, UK. He believes that most practitioners are equipped with the skills necessary to act as action researchers, 'having well-developed interpersonal skills, flexibility to respond to new situations, a degree of social entrepreneurism, a willingness to listen to alternative views, and the ability to be reflective and reflexive. The problem is in recognising and valuing such attributes in ourselves'. (Hope 1998: 25).

In some ways social researchers act out a role in their field-work and become 'performers' on a real-world stage. Any insight you can acquire into performing sincerely is therefore well worth the effort. Pam Shakespeare undertook personal research into the 'confused talk of people with dementing illnesses' and her work forced her 'to consider what, as a researcher, I bring of myself to fieldwork, and how my own performance in the field contributes to the research ...' This included examining the substance of her study using the analogy of the theatre. Introductory processes constituted the overture, followed by an examination of the role of the researcher as actor, the effects of scene stealing (i.e. imposing your own style to the point of overshadowing others, be they patients or colleagues), the role of the researcher as director and other enlightening and entertaining metaphors for the games we play in social life. Her observations make insightful and thought-provoking reading for the beginning researcher (see Shakespeare 1993: 95).

Inappropriate uses of action research

This brings us to a sensitive area, which is the appropriateness or otherwise of introducing action research in response to a particular problem. Theoretically, there should be no restrictions, and the philosophy of action research is capable of being applied anywhere.

There are a few scenarios, however, which could seriously compromise patients and practitioners and it is worth discussing these here as an early factor to be considered. Action research should never be used to:

- Drive an unpopular policy or initiative through, particularly when employers and/or those in authority have already decided on their game plan.
- Experiment with different treatments without making sure that the methodologies and protocols used meet the same criteria as other clinically based therapeutic studies.
- Manipulate employees or practitioners into thinking they have contributed to a policy decision when, in reality, it has already been made.

- Try to bring a dysfunctional team or workgroup together (whether or not they actually are dysfunctional, any doubts you may have suggest you need to examine your 'systems' first, before engaging in a time-consuming and potentially disruptive project).
- Bolster a flagging career. Action research will expose any weaknesses you may have extremely quickly.

Attempts to drive through unpopular or contentious ideas and policies are fraught with potential dangers. Employees or patients can quickly scent an ulterior motive and the loss of credibility and respect to your reputation (as well as that of your conspirators!) will soon disabuse you of any notion you might have had of trying to impose your will by stealth. Action research is only effective when educational and management systems are in place and functioning well (see Marrow 1998), and it is certainly true that without the enthusiastic support of both, few studies survive long enough to be considered worthwhile.

It could be argued, of course, that weak management or a poor educational environment is precisely why action research is needed. If this is the case, you will still need the confidence and support of key managers, educators and clinicians if you are to set up a study which is robust enough to struggle on through the difficult times in the hope of generating new ideas and structures in the workplace. Disaffection and damaged relationships do not really provide you with a solid base for your research, so that open communication and honesty are important in the first instance in helping to establish your motives as sound and ethical for good practice.

Examples of studies which have made a difference to practice, and to improving the quality of care for patients and clients, include the development and evaluation of an acute stroke care pathway via action research (Underwood & Parker 1998); an exploration into the health needs of older citizens in the community (Moyer *et al.* 1999) and a study of pain management and cultural attitudes to pain (Burrows 1997). For all the hard work, action research does bring tangible benefits, even to the hard-pressed researcher:

'Research is a confusing business encompassing lightning flashes of clarity. It is motivating with periods of despair, exhilarating but never seems to end. Even when the end does arrive there is a new beginning.'

(Burrows 1997: 86)

Why choose action research?

Having successfully convinced you that action research is extremely hard work, it now needs to be made clear when and why action research should be your preferred course of action. Choose action research when you and your colleagues are convinced that:

- you have identified an area ripe for improvement;
- you are satisfied that systems already in place are strong enough to withstand sustained enquiry;
- you feel ready to undertake a systematic, rigorous and intellectually demanding piece of work;
- you have the support (or at least the ear) of those who can make access to your research environment possible;
- you have access to the advice and support of experienced researchers, at least one of whom is knowledgeable about action research;
- your family and friends are aware of your project and they understand that you are about to become part of an additional 'research family' which will also be making demands on you; and
- your colleagues share your enthusiasm for changing and improving practice, and can see for themselves the benefits to be gained.

Whether you choose action research to assist you in critical reflection, theory development, improving practice or as an academic pursuit and the way to further qualifications (perhaps all of these), you can be sure of three things: your learning curve will be vertical, you will make many new friends and your understanding of human nature will attain new heights!

The next chapter will look at how to prepare and construct an action research proposal and how to obtain support for your proposed study.

CHAPTER 2

Preparing a proposal

Before producing a formal research proposal it is worth taking some time to establish to your own satisfaction why exactly you wish to undertake your project and what you think it will achieve. Surprisingly, not all would-be researchers take time to do this and the subsequent lack of clarity in their thinking soon emerges in a hastily cobbled together research proposal which is then rejected in its earliest stages.

One of the first things to ask yourself is 'Why me?' Where has the initiative come from? A vague feeling of unease about an issue or policy may have set you thinking. You may be at the stage of your career where you have sufficient personal confidence and work experience to feel you could make a significant and worthwhile contribution to the literature in your area of expertise. You may have enjoyed recent academic study and want to take things further. You may have read other research which strikes a chord (or is out of line) with your past experience and professional judgement. You may just be curious about a subject and want to hone your research skills as part of your professional development.

The reasons for undertaking an action research study usually derive from a feeling of dissatisfaction with an existing state of affairs. A policy or therapy is not producing the results you expected, or recent attempts to improve practice have fallen on stony ground. Practitioners who are attracted to research may see an opportunity to act as a change agent, but have misgivings about trying to tackle the problem without strategic and organisational support.

For practitioners who are also students in higher and professional education, it may simply be that you have reached the stage of maturity in your intellectual career when critiquing and working with others' research needs an added dimension, namely, the benefit of knowing for yourself what is involved in conducting and publishing research within your own field of practice.

Your reasons for getting involved are very important and may be critical to your ability to see your project to completion. It is necessary to be able to distinguish between initial misgivings or doubts based on any lack of confidence about managing your project – which are natural and to be expected – and any nagging and more serious concerns about whether you have the time and necessary commitment to follow it through. Juggling work, domestic responsibilities, a social life, study *and* research may be (for some, and with good reason) a bridge too far, and it is helpful to try and assess at an early stage your chances of doing so successfully.

This is not an attempt to discourage, or to imply that research is beyond all but a handful of elite and somehow especially gifted people. Far from it. Social research needs pragmatic thinkers who are capable of managing several tasks at once, and who refuse to be deflected from their aims by day-to-day distractions. The very fact that so many health professionals do get involved in applied research is a testimony both to their commitment and to their staying power. But this in itself is insufficient reason to think that you must get involved if you really feel in your bones that the demands on your time will be too great.

There is a clear case for practitioners being able to reflect critically on their practice and being able to critique, understand and use the research findings of others, which is documented extensively in the professional literature. The ability to take this a step further and to use the same principles to reflect *in* action on current practice in addition to examining decisions retrospectively is also, arguably, the hallmark of a professional. If this makes you feel duty-bound to get involved or guilty for your lack of previous involvement, take heart. The very notion of the practitioner-as-researcher is a relatively new development which is only now gaining ground in health care practice, largely because of dissatisfaction with the traditionally imposed model of separation between those doing the research and those upon whom research is conducted. Practitioner-researchers have a bright future if they can prove to themselves that combining the roles results in improved and innovative practice, but they cannot (yet) always depend on having the necessary support available to them locally to help them realise their professional ideals. Existing systems and institutions under fiscal pressure barely function adequately as service providers. Hence, as the research community within practice grows, it will also need to develop its own specific support networks and structures to support practitioner research, so that the kind of critical reflexivity discussed in the previous chapter is both nurtured and valued.

Therefore, if you decide to venture out as an action researcher you will need to develop an emotional toughness and resilience which will help you to sustain yourself (and, at times, your colleagues) through times that will be demanding and sometimes intellectually challenging. You will have many opportunities to ask yourself 'Just why *are* we doing this?'

There will also be times of enormous reward, particularly when, just as you were about to give up, something new or intriguing turns up. Then you find you just have to continue a little longer, and before you know it you have made significant progress. Action research is actually a bit of a tease: it has the potential to make you despair of creating a culture for change, while at the same time preparing the ground in a way you probably never dreamed was possible. Too few texts succeed in conveying the serendipitous and emotional nature of research discovery. The next section outlines the process of constructing the necessary research proposal to get you started and on your way.

Structure and content

The structure and content of your proposal will need to take account of where the initiative for the research is coming from and where you intend to conduct your research. Some employers and health authorities prefer you to fill in a proforma, or provide guidelines to help you in setting out your proposal. Clearly it is in your best interests to comply with these, but be warned that they tend to be biased towards a medical model. Thus, if your study is purely qualitative (and you do not intend to include any quantitative element in your overall design), it is unlikely that your proposal will fit neatly into the right columns.

This has implications in that any significant remove from what is expected may be treated dismissively, or taken less seriously than standard quantitative proposals, particularly in very prestigious teaching hospitals or medically dominated academic departments. This does not necessarily mean that your proposal will run into difficulty, but you should have at least an elementary understanding of what the funding agency, employer or institution is expecting (usually a randomised controlled trial!) and be able to justify your own methodological choices against those which are more familiar to members of research or ethics committees.

In the UK National Health Service (NHS) all research proposals should be approved by local research committees, as NHS Trusts are autonomous, independent organisations established by statute. Individual trusts are therefore responsible for seeing that research is conducted to a professional standard, and for ensuring that neither patients nor staff are compromised in any way by the study being undertaken. They will want to assess the indirect as well as direct effects of the study, and so you need to be prepared and able to describe what these may (forseeably) be. Outside of state funded services there may also be commercial interests that will influence the kind of research you do (i.e. the interests of insurers, suppliers and sponsors) and you will need to seek advice from the relevant member of staff.

As a matter of courtesy, it is wise to inform your line manager of any proposed research. They will want to know how it is likely to affect your role at work and your professional development, and to discuss the impact (if any) on patient care and staff workload. Try to be constructive and frank about this and be prepared to reach a compromise in order to get your manager's approval. Without it you are unlikely to get very far. Trusts or other employers will also want to see what they will get in return for their support. This is sometimes called a *research bargain* (of which more later), which is entered into when you negotiate access to your chosen research site.

Academic departments may also have their own format for outline research proposals and it will help if at this stage you can find an experienced researcher to talk you through it. In the early days before an academic supervisor is assigned to you, it is helpful to engage in free discussion about any worries you may have. In this way you may be signposted to a particular member of staff with a special interest in your subject, rather than being assigned to a particular supervisor simply because they are due to take on a new student and they are available.

All research proposals need to contain the following:

- a working title (which may be refined over time);
- a summary of what you intend to research, where you want to conduct it and who needs to be involved;
- an outline of the aims of your study and what you hope to achieve;
- an initial literature review which puts your study in context;
- details of your chosen methodology and your justification for choosing it;
- a proposed timescale, together with details of how you intend to feed back to your sponsors/employers/supervisors on progress over the time allocated;
- a consideration of the ethical issues your study is likely to generate and how you propose to deal with these;
- details of resources needed and the likely time and cost implications of involving members of staff as co-researchers;

- an idea of how you intend to report on your study and disseminate its findings; and
- details of your own professional and research background and your personal motivation for undertaking the study.

If you are preparing a proposal purely for academic purposes then there is perhaps no need to include your costings unless they are specifically asked for. If your proposal is to be directed to a funding agency, detailed costings will be a vital prerequisite to obtaining support for your work. Your professional library and, in the UK, the *Times Higher Educational Supplement* provides regular listings and contact addresses of funders. If this is your first proposal it may be prudent to seek the advice of an experienced researcher who has attracted funds before. Different agencies have different priorities, however, so take advice from them directly as to how best to undertake the formal costings part of the application procedure.

Defining your research question

A good deal of angst and worry often surrounds defining the wording of the all-important research question. If this is vague or woolly, we are warned, then the project will be in serious jeopardy.

Action researchers can take comfort that whatever your question started out as, it is unlikely to remain so for the duration of your project. Often action researchers start with an issue and before long they find themselves looking at a range of problems, all of which would make interesting avenues for study. Decisions have to be made about which avenues can be explored, given your timescale and the talents within your particular research team. They need not all be made at the beginning, however, and you should allow yourself some time to develop your thinking in response to new issues which arise.

By all means stay focused on your original question, and continue to track what has happened in relation to this all the way through. But if you find yourself worrying about whether the question you have in mind is adequate or good enough or appropriate to the task ahead of you, stop and take advice before deciding to abandon it in favour of another option. Being reflexive in your approach is about responding to changes and new ideas generated in practice and, if everyone is doing this successfully, inevitably your research question will adapt to accurately reflect what it is that your study has uncovered.

Another word of caution is offered here. You need to be able to track carefully from the beginning of your project to the point at which your personal involvement ends. It will not help to simply abandon your original question just because the data that is emerging does not fit. You need to be able to see how the threads of data and analysis are woven together, and the ways in which the data or evidence (depending on the actual data collection techniques used) has evolved in response to your initial intervention. There will be more consideration of this in Chapter 3 when we come to look at how to go about making sense of 'raw' data.

Advice is offered by Mason (1996) on general questions to ask yourself at the beginning of your study to keep you on the right track. When formulating your research question(s) you should think about the following.

- Ask yourself whether you are clear about the essence of your inquiry, and the intellectual puzzle you are trying to solve.
- Is your research question coherent? If you have asked more than one question are your questions coherent and do they add up to a sensible whole? Will everyone else understand them as you do, for example?
- Are your questions open enough to allow for the degree of exploratory study needed? Are they likely to generate further questions at a later stage?
- Are your questions original and worth asking? Remember to draw on your initial literature review.

As an action researcher you will almost certainly need to ask 'What difference is the proposed study likely to make to current thinking and practice?' Provided you have thought through and are satisfied with your answers to these questions, then your title and research question are likely to be quite robust.

If you are in doubt, then you need to go back to basics and ask yourself what it is you hope to achieve. (Sadly, 'a qualification' is not a good enough answer. It would be very difficult to justify the cost and co-researcher involvement of an action research study just to provide the researcher with letters after his or her name. There are easier, less labour-intensive and organisationally costly ways of doing this, and you need to consult your supervisor to discuss what these might be.)

Even before you attempt your proposal you may want to take soundings on the likely success of your venture in the workplace. This can involve meeting with managers, practitioners and educators, talking to people within your professional networks, your mentor and other experienced members of staff.

Action researchers sometimes choose to engage in a small-scale pilot study at this stage, whereby the stakeholders, i.e. those with a stake or interest in your research, have their say in how your study should be shaped. Key people in the workplace can make or break your study, so it is worth finding out who the professional gatekeepers are who have the influence and power to help you bring your project together.

Tierney refers to the beginning stage as 'conceiving and defining the project' and describes it as the 'thinking and reading stage of research. From a review of the literature we clarify what is already known about the topic; then decide what new research is most appropriate, relevant and feasible; and then define the project in terms of research aims'(Tierney 1997: 39). A substantive review of the literature at the beginning stage is less important in action research projects than in other types of research, for reasons which will now be explained.

Literature reviews and the action research process

In action research, searching and reviewing the literature is a continuous process conducted (where possible) and fed back to the group by all participating co-researchers for as long as the study lasts.

An initial review of the literature on the subject is usually carried out by the individual who initiates the project, for their own purposes, for the information of those supporting or funding the study and also as an introduction to the study topic for would-be co-researchers. It is important to remember that co-researchers have to be recruited into participation, and that a sound, well-written and authoritative literature review which addresses issues from both a theoretical and practice perspective is the principal means of getting people interested in your study.

Attempts are usually made to be non-hierarchical within the action research team, but in practice, particularly if undertaking a larger scale study, you will need at least two or more people to act as co-ordinators for other co-researchers.

Co-ordinators (sometimes referred to as facilitators) share responsibility for some of the deskwork associated with data collection, in collaboration with the lead researcher. Some people use the term primary researcher for the person who leads the study. You will certainly need to decide on some form of terminology or your documents and reports will be difficult to write and understand. Clearly there are issues around collaborative literature reviewing which merit closer attention, which will be discussed in Chapter 3.

In the present author's experience many existing research methods texts are frustrating to action researchers because they are not designed for the reflexive and unpredictable nature of a problem-solving approach. Even when they discuss qualitative studies generally, they do not anticipate the kind of problems action researchers experience, and this can be very isolating and alarming for the intrepid action researcher who feels they may be muddling through when all other published research appears to be straightforward.

This is probably because people tend to promote their successes over their failed attempts, and few people who have given up go on to document their experiences. This is unfortunate because it is through examining our difficulties that we learn new things. All researchers make mistakes of some kind or another, but when it comes to writing up, most people naturally concentrate on the positive aspects. When confessional accounts appear they can be very comforting, and perhaps as we grow in confidence as researchers we will be less afraid to expose our mistakes to critical review. In action research all mistakes have very direct consequences, so it is difficult to avoid being honest about these. Openness and a sense of humour are therefore essential!

Pilot studies and Delphi techniques (for example, see Williams & Webb 1994) whereby stakeholders are consulted on their views, can be very enlightening and help to direct you to key movers and shakers in your proposed research environment. They can also alert you to potential dead ends or blind alleys where your research is unlikely to receive the attention it deserves.

Pilot studies involve making a tentative small-scale exploration of your chosen topic before going on to design your substantive study. Some researchers believe that in qualitative research this is unnecessary, as qualitative methodology should be flexible enough for you to 'learn on the job' (Holloway 1997, citing Robson 1993).

Delphi techniques involve finding out who the experts are on your chosen topic and consulting them on their views as to pertinent questions for study. Gaining access to experts may not be straightforward, however, and you may need to identify a number of individuals and send them an explanatory letter and a short questionnaire. Some may express strong preferences, and you will require canny intuition if their field is a small one and affected by professional rivalries and hidden agendas. Perhaps the best advice is to do what feels right for you. No time taken to clarify and become more familiar with your subject is ever wasted, even if you ultimately do not rely on your pilot or Delphi studies in the longer term.

Undertaking a pilot study

Benefits to be gained from an initial pilot study include the following.

- Gaining valuable background knowledge and information on who is available to help you with your study.
- Acquiring a sense of how feasible your study will be.
- Getting access to practitioners and their opinions on the problem to be studied (Do they consider it a problem? If so, how do they think it should be tackled and by whom?).
- Early warning of any potential pitfalls or blocks to progress, such as staff who feel your involvement is unnecessary and unwarranted, or who may feel threatened by your study. Remember that it may not be you they feel threatened by, but low morale which is behind their negative feelings towards you.
- An idea of what your study will involve. How will you identify potential co-researchers, for example, and how are you going to go about bringing them together as a group?

Bear in mind that if you hit real snags at the pilot stages, you are unlikely to be successful in your main study. Some very innovative projects have bitten the dust simply because the early warning signals as to whether the study was workable were not taken sufficiently seriously at the beginning.

The main criteria for your longer term study are:

(1)   Is it feasible?
(2)   Is it necessary?
(3)   Is it likely to sustain everyone's interest?
(4)   Is it ethical? (for example, does it compromise anyone?)
(5)   Is it desirable? Will it add anything to current research and experience?

A pilot study should help you to identify any weaknesses in the proposal for your main study, and information from this can be used to strengthen the claims made for your study in your formal proposal. Different readers will be looking for different things in your proposal.

Managers will want to see your justification for the time, energy and financial commitment involved, while your research supervisor will want evidence of your intellectual capacity to complete the study. Your colleagues will want to have a good idea of the scope and purpose of your project, particularly if you are asking them to becoming fully involved as co-researchers. What will you be expecting of them exactly and what will it mean for them in the context of their other professional and social commitments?

Choosing a setting

Sometimes it is easiest to set up a study away from your normal workplace, because then you will not be affected by existing relationships between you and your present colleagues. The drawback is that it will take time to establish yourself as a new member of another team, and you will have to overcome your sense of being an outsider, at least at the beginning. Your knowledge of the personalities and foibles of the team members will be less reliable, although they may be less affected by old rivalries too!

Be prepared for some colleagues and managers who may express suspicion or wariness of your motives. This may only be a product of the culture in which people have been expected to work. It need not be personal and so you must take care not to view it as such. If you start out with a basic distrust of each other, it will then be very difficult to earn trust without an open and giving attitude. Outward cynicism may come from others' disappointments with either the system or their colleagues, and you will need to deal with this phlegmatically if you meet it.

Developing an ethically sensitive approach

As Lathlean has explained, positivist research emphasises theory testing, rigorous measurement and an external perspective of a single tangible reality that is governed by laws and which can be fragmented into variables, each capable of independent study. The *interpretive* tradition, with which action research is consistent, instead emphasises 'theory generation and an internal perspective on multiple tangible realities which can only be studied holistically' (Lathlean 1997: 34). The commitment to social action made by every action researcher necessarily opens them up to ethical scrutiny, including the need to be able to justify action on ethical grounds. The very act of collaborating, for example, means that we are all involved in behaving ethically, and are collectively (as well as professionally) accountable for the actions we undertake.

Gaining ethical consent for a practice-led study may be necessary, particularly when there are clear implications for patient care or treatment. Arguably, anything which adds to employees' workloads has potential implications for the delivery of care. Issues of confidentiality and anonymity in action research are also contentious because projects are often made public in order to gain support and thus participants (and their settings) are reasonably easy to identify once a report is published.

When writing up an action research study, extreme care is needed to ensure that individual participants or work cannot be identified, except where express consent has been obtained. This is much easier to say than do, and any issues which arise unforeseeably must receive attention without delay.

Research ethics usually concern issues such as the need for:

- voluntary (as opposed to coerced) participation;
- participants to have given *informed* consent;
- preventing participants and others who may be indirectly involved from becoming psychologically or physically harmed by the research;

- individuals to retain the right to withdraw from the study and/ or to retract consent;
- anonymity and confidentiality;
- accurate recording and safe management of data produced by the study;
- observation of professional and employer codes of conduct;
- adequate feedback and reporting of the study's progress; and
- mutual respect and support of co-researchers as part of a collaborative team.

Studies must be conducted within the law, and must not place co-researchers or those they work with at any physical or psychological risk. When studies are large and turnover of staff is high, consent may need to be obtained several times. It is also not uncommon for staff to want to withdraw their consent at different stages because of changing family or work commitments. Job changes, departmental changes, promotion, sickness absence and study or maternity leave can all wreak havoc with our initial cohort of participants and lead us to feel unsure as to whether collaboration is effective. Some co-researchers may find the demands on their time too great; others will worry about whether they are 'doing enough'.

It is important for the lead researcher to try to stay abreast of developments within the research environment. In the present author's doctoral study, co-researchers had the disconcerting habit of developing their teaching and interpersonal skills through the project and then being promoted very quickly. All research therefore has potential side-effects, and while you cannot always plan ahead for these, it is really important to remain aware of the undercurrents affecting your study, and to put in place remedial action when necessary.

Chapter 3 will include more discussion on recruiting and preparing co-researchers. If you find it hard to obtain consent for your study either from managers, employers or co-researchers, you may be being unrealistic in your expectations and need to review these. If you should also find consent being withdrawn early on, this requires urgent investigation to see whether the problem is due to local issues or whether the research problem you are exploring is more complicated than you thought.

Again, it would be wise to take advice from an experienced researcher if anything you plan to do has ethical implications. The statutory bodies and professional organisations for health workers can often provide helpful guidelines and managers, too, may have developed specific policies to ensure ethical research practice within your specialist area. Trades unions and patients' representative organisations can also be extremely knowledgeable and forthcoming on issues which are likely affect their members.

An area that needs careful handling, particularly in practitioner-led research, is the role of service managers and their part in the collaborative process. This is considered in more detail under 'Managing relationships' in Chapter 3.

Establishing a realistic timescale and workplan

A critical part of getting your study to run as smoothly as possible is both working to a realistic timescale and preparing a plan of work which will clearly set out both the objectives of your research and the allocation of various tasks which need to be completed.

The timescale and workplan will depend on the scale and scope of your study. For example, if you are a general practitioner who wants to assess the implementation of a new staff development policy, then six months would be a reasonable initial timescale for seeing that the plan was implemented. If you then wanted to go on to study whether the development activity was successful, this would require a more extensive time period, together with a consideration of the different methods to be employed in order to evaluate development from the perspectives of the staff involved. Should you then decide to adopt an alternative approach (on the grounds that the intervention was not as successful as was hoped for), then more time would have to be allocated and a further analysis made of the effects of that intervention, and so on.

Hence, action research is far from a short-term quick-fix approach to problems in practice. Rather it develops with practitioners and continues to challenge them to justify decisions on theories about practice *emerging from practice*, and not just what other voices in the literature advise them to do.

Let us look at another example. You are a community pharmacist wishing to rearrange the reception area of your pharmacy because the present arrangements are thought to be too public and may be discouraging patients from asking for your confidential, professional advice. Co-researchers here are those employees who assist the pharmacist and of course the general public who try to access advice and services. A period of three months might be enough to see whether more people ask for advice once the new arrangements are in place, but as you will want to compare this with the previous uptake you will probably want to plan for a fact-finding period to establish what the present uptake is. Anecdotal evidence may be enough to set you thinking about what is needed, but in order to be rigorous you also need to make strict comparisons. An action research project which purports to be rigorous will therefore rarely be completed in a short time.

You may also want to *triangulate* your methods, that is, try out various methods of data collection and compare them to see whether they point to the same (or differing) explanations. Hence, in this example you might employ a number of techniques to give you an accurate idea of the present situation, such as interviewing the dispenser and pharmacy assistants, asking patients to complete a short questionnaire (both in the pharmacy and perhaps in the neighbouring health centre), and perhaps seeking the advice of the local Community Health Council or consumer organisation. For each additional layer of people you involve, invariably your timescale will need to expand.

As new problems and issues emerge, more time is needed to deal with ethical issues, and you will need to build in to your timescale sufficient time to appraise these issues as and when they arise.

All this might lead you to conclude that it is very difficult to plan a reliable timescale at all. Action research is less 'controllable' than other research approaches and you need to expect this as a natural by-product of your research as a cyclical and reflexive process.

Putting together an initial list of tasks will help you to develop a workable plan of action, and when you have done this (usually after your pilot study stage) this should give you a better idea of the amount of time needed. When you have decided roughly how much time to give to your study, add at least another six months and you should be reasonably on target! More information about the necessary workplan also appears in the next chapter.

Action research and academia

Action research has an established pedigree in teacher education, humanistic psychology and organisational or management development. However, it has yet to be widely accepted within many of the more traditional disciplines, largely it would seem because it is based on researcher involvement in finding solutions to practice problems, an approach which some consider too subjective and open to distortion. Educational action research in particular has attracted some stern criticism because it can appear over-intricate and complex (see Robson 1993: 438–444).

Some action researchers go to the trouble of devising long and involved models or frameworks when they outline the tasks or stages involved in action research, which may be their way of planning and conceptualising their research practice. Such models may be helpful to read or they may not, depending on whether you think visually. While a sound grasp of the various stages involved in the research process is vital, models or frameworks need not be a prerequisite for successful action research.

Those preparing to undertake action research for academic credit or as part of their studies for a higher degree might also like to keep the following in mind. Action research is still actively resisted by some academic departments, perhaps because the control of events is difficult to monitor from a distance. The ethical implications of a study can be immense, and require careful and proactive management. Potential supervisors may try to discourage it for reasons they may or may not be clear about. Some will say it is too involved, too risky, too unmanageable, or too difficult to write up, when what they mean is that it is difficult and time-consuming to supervise.

Others may warn you against starting something which, for domestic or work reasons, you may not be able to finish. Conversely, some supervisors may be very enthusiastic yet inexperienced in supervising students who are using an action research approach. You need to try to steer a middle line between rushing to get involved or being frightened off unnecessarily.

For doctoral students one of the main problems academic departments have is finding a suitable external examiner (one who understands the principles of action research and who has sufficient experience of the methodology *and* your field of practice to examine you fairly). Sometimes the two qualifications are difficult to find in one person, so that you might like to see whether two external examiners would be a suitable compromise.

Remember that for all its success in health and social care (see, for example, Hart & Bond 1995) there is still a considerable way to go in persuading our traditionalist colleagues of the merits and rigour of the action research approach.

Establish, therefore, at the beginning of your study that your supervisor knows enough to guide you in the appropriate direction. Extend your personal and professional networks, especially the formal collaborative action research networks operating in recognised centres of excellence. Attend meetings and conferences on action research and try to consult as many completed action research theses and dissertations as you can. Get a feel for what is involved and ask around as to who is likely to make a suitable examiner for you. Steer your head of department in their direction when the time comes.

Not all departments are as reasonable as this, however, and some students will have to make do with whoever is both prepared to read their work and available when the time to undertake the viva (oral examination) arrives.

If on your travels you are introduced to someone who seems to have the same interests and enthusiasms as yourself, see if they might act as a mentor to you, or at the very least exchange ideas about the role of action research and their particular ways of dealing with problems as they are experienced in practice.

Some kind of psychological and emotional support will be necessary to help you through the ups and downs of your degree studies, and it is helpful to think ahead as to who your supporters will be. If you plan to be the lead or primary researcher, it is likely that your co-researchers will look to you for support at critical moments, and you want to be sure you feel able to do this when the time comes.

If the study proposed is interprofessional, large scale, or has several key aspects to it, think about and take advice on whether as colleagues you may pursue your studies jointly, with several of you following through the same study, but taking different disciplinary or theoretical strands, and then analysing it and writing it up from your own professional and philosophical perspectives. Other researchers have successfully integrated academic and professional development into their research studies (see, for example, Bamford *et al.* 1998). This takes the idea of collaboration a stage further, and is a useful model which satisfies other external demands for providing opportunities to work interprofessionally, as well as providing excellent value for money.

Work very hard, too, on always justifying your approach to your study. Check it out with other researchers and see whether your work is sufficiently grounded and an authentic account of what is going on in practice. Take nothing for granted as an action researcher and remember that the world is a gendered place, subject to unequal power relations (Maynard & Purvis 1994).

Some action researchers prefer to draw on a broad range of theories to illuminate their studies, while others choose to defend and develop a single theory or argument in greater depth.

Remember, too, that research supervision is a learning experience for your supervisor as well as for you. Get to know and understand your supervisor's ways. They have likes and dislikes and preferred ways of working and you will need to compromise over the allocation of time and how much guidance, support and feedback is necessary. Relationships with supervisors are a strangely under-reported phenomenon in the literature, although some recent texts have attempted to demystify the supervision process and provide suggestions on how best to manage the process successfully (for example, Holloway & Walker, 1999).

Mutual respect is a good basis from which to start, and clearly the ways in which supervisors are assigned has much to do with how valued people feel. If you and your allocated supervisor have nothing in common and/or fail to create that vital 'spark' between you which helps you to clarify and develop your thinking, then do something about it at an early stage. Obviously if you can choose your supervisor then this is a bonus, but give some careful thought to the reasons for your choice.

React constructively to comments made about your work but do not be persuaded into accepting someone else's opinion without being able to justify it yourself. It is part of a supervisor's role to act as devil's advocate sometimes. It is far preferable to have to justify your statements ahead of time than to flounder when the viva is under way.

Find out who is responsible for overseeing research students in your department and ask for formal written guidance on how the supervisor relationship is monitored and managed. What further help and support is available to students in addition to the supervisor relationship, for example? If you find this is a departmental weakness, either get together with other students to ask for what you need, or find another more helpful department or university. A university which does not treasure its next generation is not good enough for your trail-blazing work, so consider going elsewhere if you feel it necessary.

In the same way, departments have different philosophies and expertise, so check to see what these are and how they are likely to fit in with your own approaches to learning. Might another department be more sympathetic and knowledgeable about the resources you need? Use your professional as well as academic libraries to the full and never be afraid to ask what you may feel are stupid or naive questions. Identify key staff in the library and find out what their specialist skills and interests are. Even in large academic institutions try to develop a rapport and a good professional relationship with key staff. Resources may be stretched but, if you are realistic and reasonably patient about what you need, staff are usually pleased to be asked, particularly if it gives them the chance to use their personal expertise. Time devoted to getting to know and understand your library resources at the beginning stages of a study can pay huge dividends later on, so do not allow yourself to be rushed at the start.

Fellow students are a source of friendship and informal and social support. Develop networks and do not be tempted to treat others doing similar work as potential rivals. Enabling skills are often developed by a good peer relationship and if you begin by being open and interested then others are more likely to respond positively.

Finally, try to understand and use the language of the different worlds you encounter as a research student. The cultural practices and understandings of your workplace may not be well understood in academia, and similarly, established academics have a 'life-world' which can seem quite foreign and confusing to those of us with pragmatist leanings.

Devise some morale-boosting activities for those times when your work appears to be getting nowhere or threatens to overwhelm you, so that you can take time out without feeling guilty. Build in a reward system for yourself which acknowledges your hard work and the small (but nonetheless significant) hurdles you learn to overcome. Keep your work in perspective and do not let it define you as a person. It is only one aspect of your life and you want to enjoy it as that. There is life after your research!

CHAPTER 3

Managing action research

This chapter aims to provide an overview of the processes involved in managing a project or study based on action research. Suggestions are made concerning:

- the process of negotiating access to your chosen research site;
- recruiting and preparing co-researchers;
- managing feedback processes;
- managing the relationships which have been created by the research process;
- managing time;
- data collection and handling; and
- managing bias.

Chapter 4 will then take things a stage further by looking at the ways in which data is used to create an understanding of the phenomena you are attempting to study by virtue of the *analytic process*. To begin with, however, we need to look at the ways in which action research contributes to the overall goals of social research in order to 'locate' it both pragmatically and philosophically.

The goals of social research

Ragin describes the goals of social research as 'giving voice' to previously unheard groups in society, providing people with the means to explore and re-interpret historically or culturally significant phenomena and the wherewithal to stimulate new theoretical thinking (Ragin 1994: 83–84).

Action research can be used for all of these purposes, although it is open to multiple interpretations and to manipulation by researchers and stakeholders. Hart and Bond (1995) set out a useful typology for action research which can help researchers to clarify their thinking and values concerning the research process and the social outcomes they aim to produce.

As regards the *change process*, action research can be categorised roughly into four kinds: experimental, organisational, professionalising and empowering.

In the *experimental* type, action research is conducted as an experimental intervention which is used to test or generate theory, with the problem being solved in terms of the research aims only. This is based on the traditional view of the social sciences as being able to infer a relationship between cause and effect and thus being able to manipulate change in response to established social theories of group dynamics and group behaviour.

The *organisational* type tends to be top-down, directing change to predetermined (usually management defined) aims, with some hoped-for consensual definition of improvement. Organisational action research tends to involve external consultants and advisers in bringing about strategic change in organisations and uses group processes and systems theories to achieve the required shift in direction as the organisation responds to changes in markets and service needs (see Neumann *et al.* 1997, Barton-Cunningham 1993). The views and concerns of employees may be secondary in this kind of research to demands made centrally by those in charge or in control of the organisation.

Professionalising action research is professionally led, with the problem being studied and resolved in the interests of research based practice and professionalisation, that is, 'towards improvement in practice defined by professionals and on behalf of users' (Hart & Bond 1995: 42). Whether it is the professionals or their clients (or indeed, both) who stand to gain from this approach is, of course, open to question and interpretation.

Finally, the *empowering* type is characterised by a 'bottom-up, undetermined, process led' intervention, where the aim is to develop greater understanding of the meanings of issues and which is geared towards negotiated outcomes that take into account different vested interests (Hart & Bond 1995: 40–43, Table 3.1). The concept of empowerment is based on the assumption that society oppresses its less vocal members and leaves them vulnerable to exploitation from those with greater power and influence. The aim of empowerment is therefore to help oppressed groups to explore the nature of that oppression and to give voice, through consciousness-raising, to those who would otherwise not be heard (see Freire 1972, Gibson 1991). The empowering type of action research acts on behalf of the unheard to create a forum for voicing their concerns with a view to improving their situation and, ultimately, increasing their share of power.

From this typology it is possible to see how the different strands of action research have evolved since Lewin's day (Lewin 1948). In health care, action research has addressed issues concerning professional development and autonomy (for example, Breda 1997, Rolfe & Phillips 1997). It is also beginning to be used as a means to implement clinical guidelines and policies based on quantitative as well as qualitative assessments of therapeutic value. All approaches assume that change is possible and that the research process itself is capable of producing as well as reflecting change in real-world settings.

Action research and the change process

Generally speaking, then, it is important for action researchers to have an appreciation of change processes and to read around change theory in order to be able to recognise and be sensitive to culturally produced reactions to change. (Suggestions for further reading are provided at the end of this book.) A working knowledge of human responses – and resistance – to change can be useful when it comes to describing and analysing the nature and extent of change generated by research activity, whatever its overall aims.

In qualitative research the emphasis is on the 'human-as-instrument' (Maykut & Morehouse 1994) and so some advance warning and understanding about the transitions people make from one set of understandings to another can be an asset.

Change and transition are two very distinct processes, with change being perceived as something which happens to people, while transition is the process of letting go of one position and moving on to another (Broome 1990). Transitions may initially create shock or detachment and involve reactions of defensiveness and retreat, before the person or group comes to terms with the transition and finally acknowledges and adapts to whatever change is affecting them (Adams *et al.* 1976, Broome 1990, Fisher 1990, Fiske & Chiriboga 1990, Mason *et al.* 1991, Bridges 1996, Merriam & Yang 1996).

Being prepared for human responses to change can therefore help you as a researcher to identify what kind of action research your problem or proposed research question implies and also gives you a head start in being able to anticipate the reactions of those you approach when negotiating access to your chosen research site.

Negotiating access

Researchers must obtain permission for entry to the setting they wish to study in order to gain access to participants. Formal permission is important and protects everyone involved (Holloway 1997). Access and ethics are the two key issues likely to confront the researcher at the beginning stages of a study and are likely to remain a concern throughout (Blaxter *et al.* 1996). Blaxter and colleagues offer some useful tips on both issues to consider at the beginning of your study and some ideas on how to increase your chances of gaining access.

Some of these have already been considered in the previous chapter, for example, who the key informants are, what demands you expect to make on participants, and so on. Tips include being modest and realistic in your requests, making effective use of existing contacts and those of your manager/supervisor/colleagues. Be very clear as to what resources you will need: people, advice, documents, when and where and how. Avoid times when people are very stressed or busy and see whether you can offer those in the setting something back for their efforts (the research bargain mentioned earlier) (see Blaxter *et al.* 1996: 143).

Explain your reasons for undertaking the research and what skills you will bring to the process. Can those you involve locally use your initiative as a way of developing themselves professionally, for example? Will it enhance team working and effectiveness? What credit will those in the setting be able to take for moving your research forward and can you provide evidence of how this will be managed ethically in terms of researcher professionalism and confidentiality? What plans do you have for co-publication and involving your participants as co-researchers in the process of dissemination?

Consider also whether your request might be affected by other activities being undertaken in that area. It is not unusual nowadays for some settings to be subject to several different kinds of research activity, and not all studies can be run concurrently. You also have to avoid over-loading would-be participants as this can clearly have an impact on the time they have available to provide or manage care safely.

Local politics can be very interesting and may reveal a power struggle over whose research is the most important. Tact and sensitivity to little nuances can help you to avoid stepping on the wrong toes, and it is worth listening for the subtle cues which indicate a potential problem or stumbling block. Half-hearted support or outright resistance may not easily be overcome.

Blaxter *et al.* are comforting to read in that they surmise that 'relatively few researchers end up studying precisely what they set out to study originally' (*ibid.* 144). It is vital, however, not to give up at the first hurdle, as resistance may in fact be due to a lack of understanding or appreciation of what your research has to offer, rather than any deep-seated aversion to your study.

Remember to take local pressures into account (ask what these are if they are not obvious) and build in some coping strategies in your workplan to deal with periods of time when other priorities have to take precedence over data collection.

You may need to gain access to official documents which may be stored electronically or manually. Powell and Lovelock (1991) advise you to be realistic about the quality of data such documents will provide. Even when you have cleared access to case files or whatever it is you want to see, they suggest you remain courteous to those who have the job of looking after them and provide a full explanation of why access is necessary. Consideration of any workload implications for staff should be acknowledged openly and negotiations should be mindful of other pressures on staff (Powell & Lovelock 1991: 133).

If ultimately you are refused access to your chosen site, accept this gracefully and either revise your plans or see whether staff are prepared to suggest suitable alternatives to you. Access is something which is likely to be continually renegotiated through the action research process, as new developments or emerging issues can throw up potential difficulties and highlight conflicts of interest. Responding to these sensitively and with tact is an essential part of remaining professional and in control of your study as it develops.

Recruiting and preparing co-researchers

Once you have identified who your co-researchers need to be you will then have to actively recruit them by demonstrating why they are needed and how you would involve them in your research. The roles and responsibilities of co-researchers need to be indicated clearly in a briefing paper submitted to those interested at the beginning of the study.

Potential co-researchers may be recommended by managers, offer their services independently, be reached via professional meetings and interest groups, or suggest themselves by virtue of their pivotal position within the setting itself. To some extent they will be self-selecting in that without people at key levels or in key positions, your research will not be possible. If you can arrange to meet people as a group then you will be able to save time and thrash through the issues collectively. This can have its drawbacks, however, particularly if your research is perceived in any way as a threat to existing cherished positions or policies.

When planning your information sessions, first of all write down the key participants or 'actors' and consider what impact the research (and the intended outcome) is likely to have on their relative positions in the organisation. This will give you a clearer idea of where potential problems or resistance might lie, and also alert you to any ethical considerations. If you can, you also need to gauge internal pressures or sources of conflict operating in the setting (such as anger, resentment, jealousy) so that you can steer clear of these, or at least not provide opportunities for staff to use your research as a means of venting their existing frustrations.

If the setting is completely new to you then you will have to manage such issues one step at a time. The critical thing is to sense when co-operation is not working, and to try alternative (rather than confrontational) tactics to managing the situation from the research point of view. Few successful studies report interpersonal conflicts as a barrier to ethical research practice.

Barriers to effective (and particularly empowering) types of action research are discussed by Zuber-Skerritt (1996), who concludes that certain strategies adopted by participants can make it difficult to acquire the changes aspired to. A dependence on seniors or experts, rather than independence of thought or action, can create a problem; as can the existence of an *efficiency orientation*. Efficiency orientation comes about as a result of wanting to 'get on with the job' rather than being willing to spend time on reflection, team building and group discussion, It is an interest in short-term results in minimum time, rather than long-term effectiveness.

Interest can become too closely tied to operational issues, with participants setting less store by (and some actively resenting) the processes introduced by the lead researcher who has to guide them through the strategic planning process and the experiential learning and philosophical discussions required to bring about effective change (Zuber-Skerritt 1996: 91).

Any research which is aimed at discovery rather than confirmation or verification of others' findings needs to be both systematic and flexible. It needs to be able to respond to the unanticipated problems and detours that will almost inevitably accompany exploratory research (Layder 1993). One of the best ways of staying systematic and flexible is to treat co-researchers with respect and to acknowledge their contribution in ways which will help to reaffirm their sense of being valued at the same time as respecting their opinions or perspectives on a given situation.

Briefing papers on the progress of your research, the roles and responsibilities you expect of co-researchers and clear guidance on how you expect these roles to be managed are an important prerequisite for this. Give would-be participants the chance to express their concerns and questions and avoid at all costs any temptation to be dismissive of these. Ask them to write concerns down, if possible, and ask for suggestions from the group as to how any such potential problems might be handled. You are setting a precedent for how you intend to conduct your study as a whole.

Any group of co-researchers (and particularly larger groups) will have support needs of some sort, and you will need to think about how these can be met within your anticipated resources. If your study is small-scale and located within a single site then regular meetings of the group may be conducted at a convenient time. Messages between participants and questions needing an answer can be managed by a simple message-box located in a central position which group members can use as appropriate. Ground rules concerning the time required to respond to queries and precautions needed to maintain confidentiality need to be set at the beginning. Agreement also needs to be reached as to who is to take responsibility for certain tasks (of which more later, when we look at data collection techniques).

Personal as well as social and strategic support may be also be needed, particularly if your research touches on emotional or sensitive issues. Studies involving care and patients directly may well have emotional consequences for practitioners and patients and it is important that these are addressed within the ethical considerations outlined in your original proposal. Not all of these may be foreseen, of course, and it may be necessary to take external and professional advice from others in order to deal with any fall-out from them. Practitioners' codes of professional conduct can be very helpful, as can involving more experienced researchers and supervisors who have personal experience of managing ethical dilemmas in practice.

Critical incident analysis is a useful technique for helping practitioners to reflect on past events, particularly in personal or group discussions, but they can represent a potential minefield in terms of patient as well as professional confidentiality. Co-researchers may need guidance from others with specialist knowledge and expertise if there is any suggestion of compromising (or inadvertently having compromised) the usual rules of client and researcher confidentiality. This can be challenging, particularly if disclosure involves any suggestion of whistle-blowing or accusations of misconduct or negligence in the workplace. Should an incident occur which does risk any of the above during the conduct of your study, document your situation carefully (avoiding potentially litigious statements) and take professional advice as to how you may proceed with caution.

Much of what goes on in your study will be straightforward – even mundane – and not every researcher will unwittingly expose poor practice or face an ethical dilemma. It is important to retain a sense of proportion, and to be clear about where co-researcher involvement in research begins and ends, a contentious subject which taxes all research communities.

Sharing philosophy and values

The need to discuss *philosophy* and *values* within your new-found research community is a vital developmental stage in the research process. Having made some headway on what you feel your own beliefs and orientations are concerning the value of research, your contribution as a professional and the aims of your proposed study, you are now in a position to see whether your co-researchers share your views and, if not, how and why they differ.

Inevitably all research communities and settings will reflect the cultural attitudes and values of their participants. All that is necessary in action research is that co-researchers agree with the key principles of action research, and that they are committed to improving practice through practitioner-generated change. Those who are against the aims of action research, for example, those who believe participants should work only to directives and instructions from above, would have a problem adjusting to the democratising effects of an action research culture on their organisation.

Personal and professional values may also reflect a wide range of opinions and it is important to be sensitive to the history behind people's personal beliefs and understandings. Often it is relationships which help us to make most sense of these.

Managing relationships

Relationships involve predictable sequences of actions such as shared activities, ways of making decisions, responding to mutual demands and emotional expression. It is primarily through relationships that people come to be able to anticipate each others' perceptions and understandings (Dallos 1996). Developing shared understandings and working towards mutual goals therefore depends on the extent to which we are able to explore our mutual understandings. Action research requires co-researchers to make their professional and personal values explicit so that explanations for events can be traced back to the different constructions and understandings individual co-researchers bring to the study, together with an appreciation of how interactions are affected by cultural norms.

Conflicts can emerge when personal and professional values diverge, or when adherence to one compromises the other and presents the practitioner with a dilemma. Some clarification of values is then needed in order to identify best courses of action. Values clarification can be undertaken in groups (focus groups are particularly helpful for this), and through direct discussion between colleagues in practice. When a problem in practice is still being clarified prior to devising a solution, sometimes after intensive discussion it turns out not to be a problem after all, but rather a question of perception and interpretation.

When practitioners come together to discuss a problem they often touch on a range of potential explanations, and after discussion has taken place, some may change their views, others may hold trenchantly to their original positions, but all will be aware of different perspectives on the same problem. Action research takes advantage of this kind of discussion to clarify issues of central concern, and to flag up points of contention between opposing views.

This debate and reworking of the central concepts and issues relating to your research is a continuous process which goes on in a cyclical fashion as you implement your proposed change and then record its effects. Devising any new way of working poses a challenge to any system and you will need to develop and maintain good relationships with those involved through both bad times and good. Everyone will have a unique outlook and opinion on both the project and your involvement in it, and will go through peaks and troughs of emotion as they discard old habits and try to learn new ones.

The easiest action research projects to implement are those where practitioners involved have despaired of existing practices and are desperate to see the situation improved. If the change involves a corresponding increase in workload then co-researchers need to be forewarned and need to be able to communicate this to others who are likely to be affected in a positive way. Having negotiated access to the site generally, it is then critical that you do not overlook those who operate on the fringes of your study, technically speaking, but who nevertheless have influence and legitimate reasons for wanting to be kept informed.

Locality managers, specialist, visiting and peripatetic staff may or may not express interest, but if they do then include them in your study by explaining its aims and asking for their views. Sometimes it takes an onlooker or someone who is involved on an occasional basis to spot the shortcomings in systems and procedures and they may be able to provide you with a new perspective.

Be aware of who the stakeholders are in your organisation are and be ready to respond to their expressions of interest, but also be wary of any manipulation of your study. If you find your work taking an unexpected turn, or you appear to have acquired a different status or new and unanticipated responsibilities (one action researcher unwittingly found themselves 'saving' a community hospital, having undertaken a small-scale study on palliative care!), try to establish how this has happened and gently remind those responsible as to what you can do realistically under the auspices of action research.

Small-scale localised studies can sometimes have their impact exaggerated (perhaps to boost someone else's profile) and this can lead to problems for co-researchers who are in the front-line of local politics. It also raises expectations of what your research can achieve and these can then be difficult to live up to when it comes to disseminating your findings.

Some researchers like to keep a card index file of 'significant others' involved in their research. This can include co-researchers, relevant contact numbers, role details, and a few lines as to their part in the research process. Occasional contributors and key informants can also be added and then returned to when you need to clarify a point or observation. As the research progresses more names are added to the file and particular expertise or concerns can be noted on individual cards as 'data' in its own right. This is helpful in getting a measure of how your research has evolved over time. Do remember to date additional information, however, or when it comes to collating and analysing your data you will be unable to trace your 'decision trail' of new ideas as they have emerged. This has the potential to lead you up blind alleys and puts you at risk from muddled thinking, a point we will return to below when we look at data management and analysis.

Relationships between co-researchers can be nurtured by regular contact both in writing and in person. Group meetings can take place both formally and informally and no harm will be done to your research by turning them into social occasions. You will need to set some ground rules early on about mutual expectations and confidentiality, however. Disclosure of sensitive information can become a part of these sessions, and you need to reach agreement on what can and cannot be repeated or referred to elsewhere.

Grey areas can occur when practitioners or patients disclose information which then requires remedial action. This is where large-scale studies have a distinct advantage in that co-ordinators or key workers then create a forum for discussing and finding solutions to any ethical dilemmas which arise. In smaller scale studies you may have to rely on your own professional judgement and intuition on how to manage the situation. For students undertaking research degrees there can be a problem in divulging confidential information to supervisors as a third party. It would be helpful if you discussed this possibility at the beginning of the study and prepared a contingency plan on what to do should such a problem arise.

Other areas of potential concern regarding relationships lies in acknowledging the contribution made by co-researchers and in recognising what is a reasonable expectation in terms of their time and personal commitment. Some participants may exchange telephone numbers and agree to meet or talk out of work hours; others will see this as an unnecessary intrusion. Be clear about this from the beginning to avoid potential misunderstandings. It can also be hard when a committed co-researcher decides to withdraw from a study. They do not have to give a reason for this and they should not be put under pressure to stay. Occasionally there will be a good reason for the lead researcher to suspect that something is amiss locally and this may need further sensitive investigation.

Relationships which also need to be considered are those concerning your sponsors, your immediate colleagues (who may or may not be directly involved) and of course friends and family.

When you become very involved and busy with your study inevitably other interests and demands may slide down your list of priorities. Naturally you may meet some resistance to this and you may begin to feel guilty for not being able to meet all the demands made on you. Researchers with family responsibilities can be hit particularly hard, and some difficult choices may have to be made over how to (and whether you are prepared to) ration your time. It is unlikely that you will be able to meet the demands of academic study as well as your professional commitments without some regular intrusion into life at home. If friends and family resent this then do think very carefully before committing yourself. It would be hard on you personally to have to withdraw from your studies later on, particularly if you have staked further promotion or career development on its successful completion.

Little guidance appears to be offered to students or professionals as to the workload such a study presents. Professionals undertaking doctoral studies have to make the greatest commitment, and it may boil down to a lifestyle decision. Much depends on how important your career and working life is to you and what your plans are for the future. A recent straw poll of part-time doctoral students who were working full-time estimated the extra time needed to study at roughly twenty hours a week. This is clearly a huge chunk of leisure time over several years. One student had taken nine years, with breaks, to get to the submission stage.

Master's level studies and projects undertaken for a first degree or postgraduate diploma may not take as many months or years but they will still require a considerable number of dedicated hours of study and writing up time.

A localised small-scale study undertaken as a professional initiative will be much more manageable on a personal level and may not have to involve out of hours work at all except for some time reading around your subject. Be prepared to take advice on this.

Sponsors tend to figure large at the beginning and at the reporting stages of your study, and it is a good idea to keep in touch regularly concerning your progress if this is appropriate and in keeping with their usual practice. Funders of large-scale studies need to be kept up to date with your costs and any modifications to your original plans, and will want you to be able to demonstrate how you have managed the resources available to you.

Some sponsors demand more of their researchers than others, and depending on their own agendas they may try to have more influence over your work than you feel comfortable with. The issue of who 'owns' research and intellectual copyright is receiving more attention than previously, with some universities employing full-time staff whose job it is to develop intellectual ideas and patent them where possible. Be clear about your position and rights on this from the beginning if you can. This will be discussed again in Chapter 4 when we look at the publication and dissemination of your findings.

Managing correspondence is also a task which can get the better of action researchers. Try to establish a time and a routine for attending to this as demands for help and information from interested people outside of your own research can be quite overwhelming, particularly if you are the first to actively research in a new area. Disappointment and resentment can inadvertently be created when you are not able to get back to everyone as you have promised, and it is better to refuse and explain your reasons politely than to promise and then forget when you have other demands on your time.

Managing time

Time budgeting is one of those ideas which can look much better on paper than it feels in reality. Management guru, John Adair, suggests making good use of 'committed time', that is time that you have set aside specifically for dealing with the paperwork associated with your research. He uses the example of Marks & Spencer, where a campaign was launched to reduce paperwork. The critical question asked was 'Will the business collapse if we dispense with this form or card?' One of the cornerstones of the 'war on paper' was trusting the management of information to key workers and supervisors, rather than relying on paper controls. Another key principle was the idea of 'sensible approximation', or 'close enough' as opposed to absolutely accurate information (see Adair 1988 for further tips).

Strictly speaking it is hard to apply advice on office management to research activity, as you need to be able to see and demonstrate how your data has affected your decisions over time. The general principles still hold good, however, in that any documentation and paperwork you devise should be sufficient to the task and not unnecessarily crowded with detail or trivia.

If you can leave at least half an A4 side blank for comments from co-researchers on the user-friendliness of your documentation, they will often have suggestions as to how to manage it better. It can be extremely helpful to pilot or test your early documentation with co-researchers to get a good idea of how well it lives up to the job it was designed to do. Too little space and insufficient flexibility are common problems with record-keeping and it is helpful if you can devise a system which can be modified as your study develops. Should your methods of collecting data change you may need to revise your workplan and build in new documentation which takes into account any changes made.

The principle of delegating work to others is also a good one and can be very motivating, but you need to take care not to overload your co-researchers and to discuss your requests in advance with them rather than taking their consent for granted.

Health professionals are generally excellent time managers, having learnt the habit through necessity and experience. Data collection is a very labour-intensive process, however, and requires skilful handling if it is to stay manageable, both in the workplace and at research 'headquarters', wherever that is.

For a few lucky people this is dedicated office space made specifically available for the purpose, while for others it may be a converted loft space or garage or the corner of a room at home. Not everyone needs to go this far, however, and with careful planning you may get away with a few cupboards in the corner of a store room. (Do remember to label your boxes carefully, however, or your precious data might be sacrificed to someone else's war on paper!) This brings us to the nub of action research, the collection, handling, storage, transcription and analysis of data in relation to your study.

Data collection and management

Participation in action research is thought to be most effective when it:

- allows people to become actively involved;
- enables them to perform significant tasks;
- provides support for people as they learn to act for themselves;
- encourages the development of plans and activities which participants are able to accomplish by themselves; and
- deals personally and directly with participants rather than via their representatives or agents (Stringer 1996: 32).

Data collection and management therefore needs to take into account the resources and skills available within the research environment. Additional information and training in data collection techniques may be necessary and the responsibility for providing and/or arranging these usually rests with the lead researcher.

Action research is only one of forty different types of qualitative research (identified by Tesch 1990: 58 and listed in Dey 1993: 2). The relevance and applicability of any particular procedure therefore depends entirely on the data to be analysed and the particular purposes and predilections of the individual researcher (Dey 1993: 2).

Let us consider whether action research has particular distinguishing characteristics which make some forms of data collection more appropriate than others. Given that action research in health care tends to take place in the field, that is in locations associated with or managed by health care providers and related educational and service institutions, considerations over which data collection methods are most suitable could begin with an initial assessment of local skills and experience.

Professionalisation strategies in health care education in recent years have actively promoted a research culture, and even if practitioners have no hands-on experience of the conduct of research, most are research aware and have opinions and ideas on favoured methods and approaches. It is usually helpful to sound out your co-researchers at an early stage to see whether they have any strong preferences or dislikes.

Action researchers need methods which are:

- practical;
- feasible within the time available;
- flexible enough to move with changing priorities;
- straightforward to record and collate; and
- open to collaborative analysis.

Practical data collection means limiting the documentation and paperwork needed to the minimum required for the job. Feasibility depends on local organisational priorities and on the facilities available for storing and collating material. Consideration needs to be given to the amount of physical handling of data involved, and the number of people who will have access to it and be expected to read, transcribe and analyse it. Large-scale studies can involve sharing data across several sites and extra care needs to be taken to see that confidentiality is maintained and that none of your data is mislaid because of misunderstandings between colleagues over who has responsibility for what aspect of its management.

A clear line also needs to be drawn between primary and secondary sources of data. *Primary data* refers to information collected or produced as a consequence of the research process, for example, interview transcripts, completed questionnaires, scripts from focus group work, the minutes of relevant meetings, tapes or recordings made during the data collection period. *Secondary data* usually refers to relevant reports, existing published research, policies, articles and documents or guidelines which inform your research but which have not been produced by your co-researchers as part of your own research. This, too, needs to be read, analysed, stored and accounted for, and you will need to determine early on how both these kinds of data are managed and looked after at different stages of your study.

Great significance is attached to the meanings and cultural validity of concepts and ideas in action research. Your choice of data collection method should be influenced by which methods you and your co-researchers feel have the best chance of eliciting the thoughts and ideas of the people involved and the significance to them of what you are studying. You need to understand the context of your study and the social understandings which inform or influence that context. There is also the 'helicopter' view to be considered: that is, what are the structural influences at work, and how do people respond to the different power and gender relations operating within their social milieu?

Does your study have any political implications for participants, for example, and will this influence the kind of information they feel able to disclose or the behaviour and feelings they feel safe in exploring? What are their perceptions of the research process itself? Do they, for example, believe that your study will ultimately change anything, and if not, why not? And what implications does this have for the methods you choose?

Techniques for acquiring data

Techniques used to acquire data in health care action research are listed as follows:

- interviews;
- surveys;
- policy and/or documentary analysis and policy review;
- group discussion and clarification of values;
- critical incident analysis;
- comparison of case studies/analysis of casework;
- comparison of outcomes related to policy or treatment interventions;

- discourse (conversation) analysis; and
- critical reflection via practitioner diaries, learning logs, learning contracts etc. (i.e. *policy innovation and evaluation using all of the above to inform 'action'*).

Proposed methods and techniques need to be chosen to suit those involved in carrying it out and the cultural norms affecting their usual ways of working. The setting of an operating theatre would clearly suggest different opportunities and constraints to that of the home care settings of clients with learning disabilities. When you select which methods to use you need to take full account of the way information is usually managed in that setting and whether your method will be practical within its confines.

By taking advantage of existing arrangements you are more likely to encourage active participation. Long, involved interview schedules and in-depth questionnaires have their place, but this is often later in an action research study when you have had an opportunity to see what the most important concepts and issues are. Too intensive a methodological approach in the beginning stages can only bog you down in lengthy periods of transcription which, if done straightaway can lose your study valuable momentum, and if left to for later can leave everyone feeling over-burdened and anxious because they are failing to keep up.

When and if you decide that it is appropriate to conduct more in-depth interviews or group work, give people plenty of warning, and be extremely clear about what the process will involve, where it is happening and how long it is likely to take. If you are a research student, see whether you can sit in as an observer on someone else's study initially so that you can get an idea of how long a process takes. You will also need to take co-researchers' or participants' personal and domestic needs into account. Take soundings on the best or usual venues and facilities available locally and on the timings which are likely to attract the greatest number of interested participants. Bear public holidays and other busy periods in mind when setting your dates and remember to thank those who attend for their support, both personally and in writing.

Not all potential pitfalls are obvious even to seasoned researchers. A good example of this is the company which claimed to run focus groups professionally and which invited members of the public to discussion evenings in the homes of 'hosts' employed by the company. The idea was to create a comfortable and homely environment which helped participants to offer their opinions freely and without inhibition. As a 'silent observer' the present writer was not permitted to, and had to sit mute in the corner while the study was 'skilfully' conducted by the facilitator. Unfortunately the host had placed tape recorder, drinks and snacks on one table, so that when the tapes were transcribed only the odd muffled syllable could be heard over the sound of noisily munched nuts and crisps. An otherwise excellent and very valuable three hours of data collection was consigned reluctantly (and expensively) to the dustbin. The moral is therefore to pay attention to detail and to keep a watchful eye open for the little irritations that can nevertheless threaten a study's welfare.

Read as much as possible around different techniques (see 'Further reading' for useful introductory texts) and choose only those that you are personally comfortable with. You will have to motivate others to keep going at times and need to be convinced yourself that a particular technique is appropriate and workable for you.

Spend time observing others where possible and reading through the methodological discussions written up in other similar studies to get a feel for which methods will suit your particular subject and setting. Conversely, do not discount a method because of a few criticisms, as no method is perfect and all have their particular advantages and drawbacks.

Learn the art of critiquing a study so that you can acquire the necessary antennae for recognising flaws in the overall design of a study (such as the use of inappropriate data collection methods), rather than worrying about minor hitches in data collection which most action researchers experience from time to time.

As a general rule, choose methods which encourage co-researchers to challenge their current thinking and assumptions and which do not just allow them to confirm their present opinions. They need to be able to justify their thinking and their decisions and to see possibilities for new alternatives in response to old problems. Questions and probes will need to be based on your own reading of their situations informed by your initial literature review, and some tact and diplomacy may be called for in order to address potentially sensitive or dyed-in-the-wool practices and beliefs.

Preparing your workplan

An effective workplan records the tasks needed in order to collect your data. Your overall design should enable you to draw up a list of data collection tasks so that these can be assigned in turn to the co-researchers who have agreed to undertake them. Your workplan should include details such as the date by which such tasks should be started and completed, and who will *personally* be responsible for returning the necessary documents or completed sets of data to you. Some researchers devise special collection points and visit these regularly to pick up information, completed data and any queries relating to data collection that require speedy attention.

As part of their own personal and professional development co-researchers (and especially the lead researcher) might want to keep a research diary, which not only allows them to follow the workplan through its various stages, but to which they can add memos or personal reflections on the data collection process itself. This can be extremely insightful, particularly when it comes to analysing individual items or groups of data and helps to keep the research *context sensitive*.

Workplans should be drawn up in close consultation with co-researchers except in very large-scale studies. This approach would be too lengthy and unwieldy in large-scale projects and a better approach is to obtain agreement from co-researchers to key principles (for example, to undertake two hours a week of data collection) and then to allocate tasks on the basis of locally identified expertise or preference. Everyone involved will need to make the most of their assertiveness skills so that no-one harbours resentment or feels they are taking on an unfair share of the work. Again, try to be responsive to local demands and pressures.

Provide copies of the workplan to all co-researchers and remember to update it regularly. This will encourage everyone to stay on target and give them a sense of the study's progress. Problems will also be spotted quickly if you stick to this, as any bottlenecks or obstacles will soon become obvious and you can then modify your methods to suit local conditions and developments. Keep at least one (preferably two) copies of the original workplan and each revision and you will have an immediate template for writing up the methodological discussion part of your report or study. You will also have a better chance of seeing where you are in relation to your overall timescale and a more accurate idea of whether you have succeeded in meeting your long-term objectives.

Collaborative literature reviewing

Brainstorming is the best way of getting the collaborative literature review process off the ground. You can do this with a willing band of co-researchers, but also with your research supervisor and other colleagues.

When issues of interest or relevance develop into central ideas and *concepts,* try to develop these further by asking critical questions about them. What do such concepts mean to different individuals, how are they interpreted by different 'actors' within your setting, can they be manipulated by one group in order to bring about a certain kind of behaviour in others? How is information managed within your setting and by whom, and does this have any bearing on how people respond to your central research question or the issue being studied?

Key concepts and ideas can then be read around in order to construct a *policy analysis,* or to develop further conceptualisations and critical constructs. How do people build their individual and personal social realities and then come to rebuild them as members of groups, communities and societies? What is written about these processes both in the literature we are most familiar with, and by critical writers and observers outside of our immediate disciplines and areas of expertise?

Try to share out the reading equitably and do not be afraid of taking on new ideas. Research can be viewed as a glorified detective story, concerned in a sense with the self-same mysteries and challenges that originated with the ideas and processes of social change. Conan Doyle, the celebrated creator of the archetypal detective, Sherlock Holmes, showed that the most enjoyable detective stories concerned themselves not only with crime but with the challenge of solving intellectual problems and stretching the powers of human deduction to their very limits (Alasuutari 1998: 2).

When managing a collaborative review you need to avoid duplication and keep overlap to a minimum, so that not everyone wastes time searching for and bringing back the same articles. Begin by identifying a few key texts or authors in the field and do a little 'ancestry' literature searching, i.e. reading through references and cross-references to other articles.

The golden rule for all intrepid literature reviewers is to befriend the specialist librarian for your subject in the first instance. Some libraries will undertake a literature search on your behalf but they will still need your help in establishing key words and concepts to ensure your search is sufficiently refined.

Ask co-researchers to sound out and report back on any new ideas or novel ways of looking at the literature and when you have a few spare moments see what these can add to existing debate and opinion on the subject. Do the same issues/concepts/ideas keep coming up? Are there any which keep coming up in practice but which do not appear to be acknowledged in the established literature? Keep careful note of this when it happens as it may be a useful 'analytic' clue when it comes to writing up, or in identifying stakeholders who may find your study helpful at the dissemination stages.

Label and store files of articles in a central location so that all co-researchers can refer to these as necessary. Copies can be made for personal study, but you should note and observe the copyright licensing agreement which applies to your particular institution.

Library staff can advise on this and details of what is permissible can usually be found close by the photocopiers in the library and at work. Co-researchers may want to use their action research experiences to write their own essays, journals or articles and this can be a wonderful morale-booster for the study, particularly in the middle stages of research when ideas need to be clarified and arguments reworked.

Literature reviews are a summary of your reading and thinking around a subject. They are in many ways less important in an action research study than in other research because your focus is on your intervention into a particular situation. Literature reviews therefore provide solid background for the context of your study, but they tell only a limited part of the story.

The real narrative lies in how you as co-researchers analysed and interpreted the raw data which emerged in response to your intervention and what you ultimately *did* with the analysis in the interests of improving or changing practice. The skills you and your co-researchers bring to this are ultimately responsible for demonstrating to your peers and other interested consumers of your study whether it is *culturally valid*. Is yours an accurate and meaningful account of what happened? Are your findings believable and trustworthy?

Making sense of raw data

Raw data refers to the mass of information you gather as you conduct your study. Unlike qualitative analysis in non-action research, it is not a question of putting it all together in one place and sorting it into appropriate categories for analysis. The *analytic process* in action research begins from the moment you start to develop your original research question. Every activity thereafter is part of a continuous process of analytical refinement, both of the problem you are attempting to solve and the intervention or innovation you have introduced to tackle the problem. Analysis is grounded and explicitly tied to the context in which your study takes place.

For researchers trained or brought up on conventional methodological approaches this is a significant departure from usual practice. The objective in action research is not to distance oneself from the data but to become immersed in it and to understand it from the perspective of participants who are trying to resolve or improve a problematic situation.

A common question from those new to action research is 'How then do you avoid researcher bias?' In order to answer this we need to delve deeper into the philosophical underpinnings of action research and examine to see where it fits into the theoretical paradigms which inform social research generally.

The positivist paradigm has already been discussed at some length. Alternatives to this are those of *interpretivism* and *critical social theory*. Harper and Hartman (1997) helpfully outline these as part of a discussion on the philosophy, values and assumptions affecting nursing and midwifery research. Their descriptions are represented in Table 3.1.

Action research is firmly rooted in the third paradigm of critical social theory because it firmly rejects the positivist view and, while recognising and acknowledging the interpretivist view, seeks to build on this by taking it a stage further. Interpretivist research recognises our capacity to construct or build our realities socially, but it does not *by itself* enable us to challenge any of the inequities or oppressive influences we might experience in our social world.

It provides an explanation but not a solution to the problems we encounter. Problems require action to be taken in order to make improvement possible. Research based on critical social theory requires researchers to take an inherently critical stance. The aim is to make those involved aware of what prevents them from overcoming their problems or realising their chosen goal. What processes or attitudes or ways of working create barriers to effective progress and what can be done to raise the consciousness of individuals towards the kinds of political or social action which can help them to achieve their aims? This kind of empowering or emancipatory research seeks to involve people in making their own decisions with a view to creating a fairer and more just society.

Table 3.1 Philosophical approaches to research.

Research paradigm	Researcher assumption
Positivism	There is an objective reality that exists independently of the observer, where phenomena are driven by natural laws that are accessible to observation and management.
Interpretivism	Reality is mentally constructed and is socially and culturally based. Knowledge is viewed as being constructed in a social and historical context.
Critical social theory	Perceptions, social and personal truths are constructed socially, so that an understanding of social and power structures (race, class, gender) must inform theories about social life. All knowledge is seen as subjective and open to manipulation.

Adapted from Harper & Hartman 1997: 19

Action research participants are therefore not seen or described as subjects upon whom research is conducted, but as active participants in discovering, describing and counteracting any forces which have a damaging effect on them and which disadvantage certain sectors of society and render them vulnerable.

It would be hard to claim the moral high ground for action research simply because it is philosophically based on critical social theory. All research is open to potentially corrupt influences and ulterior motives. Action research can claim, however, to be a more democratic approach to research, however, because of the openness of its methodology and its relative transparency when compared to more traditional top-down non-participative studies. Not all action research is based on this emancipatory model, but most share the principles of being educative and remaining socially aware of others' motives and actions as part of the problem-solving process.

All action research studies can be fairly said to share a common bias, however, because they are committed to changing an existing situation. The research environment at the end of the intervention will not be the same as it was before. All change involves an examination of human values and, wherever these are examined, human preferences, fears, wishes, anxieties, goals, motivations and ambitions all play a part. It is inherently biased towards social action, then, as opposed to being merely descriptive in nature.

The important thing to remember is that while such bias is an explicit and accepted feature of action research, individual and group biases do need to be accounted for carefully and their effects measured in such a way as to make their contribution to the debate meaningful and understandable to the outsider. When reading an action research study, the reader should be given a clear account of not only what happened as part of the problem-solving, but also who enacted it and why. What motivated them and how were their actions perceived by co-researchers and others affected by the problem being studied?

Researcher bias in action research is not something to be sterilised or 'controlled out', rather it is a phenomenon in its own right which is allowed to grow and develop organically, so to speak, fed and watered by the care taken to see that the opinions and values of co-researchers are heard, valued and accounted for. This does not mean that all opinions are given equal weight, as this would soon descend into a kind of cultural relativism whereby all actions were considered equally 'good' or reasonable. On this basis, our thinking would soon become muddled and circular, with no-one being able to decide on the right course of action. This would achieve a kind of political gridlock or stasis which prevents us from moving on.

At some point *value judgements* have to be made and proposed courses of action decided upon, based on critical thinking and a rational justification as to why it should be the action of choice. Having considered the possibilities and options for future action, and clarified their values as to what their ultimate goal actually is, co-researchers analyse their problem-solving activities using tools specially developed for this purpose.

Validity in action research therefore rests on whether the published study is true to the beliefs, values and aspirations of those who originally conducted the research. The means of ensuring this as far as humanly possible is considered in Chapter 4 when we look at both the analytic process and the tasks involved in writing up the analysis into a formal account of the study.

CHAPTER 4

Writing a valid account

This chapter brings us to the most challenging part of action research: process evaluation and the transformation of your data analysis into a readable and effective report and/or authoritative piece of academic writing.

There are several ways of tackling data analysis in qualitative research, but not all of them are suitable or appropriate to the particular collaborative nature of the action research process. One of the most enjoyable and productive ways of analysing data and then moving on to identify key issues for inclusion in your final report/thesis/dissertation is to treat the whole process as a learning exercise, where co-researchers work together to provide a comprehensive and credible survey of the study undertaken.

Any qualitative analysis begins with a common goal: to understand more about a phenomenon of interest (Maykut & Morehouse, 1994: 121). Action research has the potential to do much more than this, however, as it:

- identifies a problem;
- explores the nature of the problem;
- suggests possible solutions based on co-researchers' analysis and interpretation of the problem; and
- generates theories about problems based on practitioner experience.

Co-researchers in health care action research collect data based on their initial reading and ideas. As new data emerges to challenge existing assumptions made by researchers, working hypotheses are then developed and tested out in practice to see whether they are successful in improving the situation or problem under scrutiny.

The process of qualitative data analysis is fundamentally a non-mathematical analytical procedure that involves examining the meaning of people's words and actions (Maykut & Morehouse 1994). Once a significant amount of data has been gathered, it needs to be scrutinised for concepts and ideas which illuminate or tell us more about the problem being studied. (This can relate to different influences: people, policies and structures.) Forums need to be set up to discuss and debate issues raised by the initial investigation and any subsequent data collection.

Data processing

All data has to be processed. If the volume of data collected is great then it will have to be divided, labelled and distributed to co-researchers to analyse, having first of all been assessed for any privacy obligations, that is, whether some data is so sensitive it needs to be kept confidential to the individual researcher who has gained access to it. As the data will take many forms, a rough reading of it initially should determine whether all or only some of the data is worth transcribing. Some parts may not be very intelligible or legible but nevertheless should still be kept safely. It may be necessary to refer back to your original sources in the future, and nothing should be discarded without very careful thought.

Having decided on what is ultimately usable, the data should then be transcribed (preferably typed) and photocopies taken so that analysts may feel free to make notes alongside points of interest. Some transcribers leave a wide margin to one side of the transcript for just such a purpose. You may decide to keep data from different sites completely separate from each other, or alternatively, you may split it into batches on the basis of the method used (for example, all interview transcripts from all sites being kept together). Some form of distinctive and consistent marking or colour coding of transcripts will be needed to ensure that they can be traced back accurately to their source. Formal analysis begins as soon as information is processed, so that everything that has been written or said about the action research problem or question becomes a potential item for analysis.

For information on the use of computers to do analysis, see Dey (1993), Tesch 1990 and Webb 1999.

For political reasons a few studies may not get any further than the exploratory stage. It may be that a decision was made not to intervene or change policy in any way, or that collaboration had to be abandoned for other, more pragmatic reasons. Analysis will then be limited to the exploratory stages of the study and to an interpretation of why it was unable to progress.

If this is the case, it is still vital to go through with analysis and writing up, as exploratory studies can provide an invaluable source of information for other researchers who may be anticipating or undergoing a similar experience. Such studies also tell us a great deal about the context we are trying to research and so should not be sidelined or considered inferior in any way to more extensive research.

Assuming that your work gets as far as exploring and defining a problem, your analysis begins with the first trawl of transcribed data. The ways in which you have recorded your data will have implications for the kinds of analysis you undertake. Ideally, data should have been recorded in a format which facilitates analysis (Dey 1993). The double bind for inexperienced researchers is that until you have used and become familiar with different methods yourself, it is difficult to recognise the limitations of particular methods for your particular topic area or research setting. There may be highly context-specific reasons as to why one method should be favoured over another, not all of which can be planned or accounted for in advance.

Extensive reading and discussion around data collection methods is advisable, and if you are offered training in research methods, take it up. Too often researchers are criticised for not taking enough advantage of the expertise available to them from colleagues, so if you know of someone with personal experience of your chosen methodology see if they will be prepared to discuss the pros and cons with you in advance.

Principles of collaborative analysis

Collaborative analysis requires co-researchers to:

- share the work involved in analysing data equally;
- respect each others' special areas of skill and expertise;
- validate their work (through recognised validation techniques);
- reflect on their own research practice and recognise the impact they have as individuals on the research setting;
- listen carefully to each other, to challenge any underlying assumptions and to seek justification for these; and
- maintain a collegial and supportive atmosphere based on mutual respect and trust.

Few real-world research environments are necessarily conducive to such principles, however, and considerable give and take on the part of co-researchers will be needed. Assertiveness skills are extremely helpful in collaborative projects and if you or your co-researchers lack confidence in this area, see whether you can read up on them and rehearse them as part of the warm-up to support group meetings. A sense of humour is vital in any case, and you may need to devise a few 'ice-breakers' for the times when you come together as a group. Tiredness and pressure at work can often be relieved by collegial support and occasionally you may find a group meeting turns into a therapy session for beleaguered practitioners who need to have their emotional batteries recharged! It is important to keep a focus on your research but to be mindful that other pressures can be useful discussion points in relation to the problem being studied.

Action research and 'reliability'

In the conventional social scientific approach 'reliability' is an indicator of how well you have carried out your research, the criteria for success being whether a similar study in a similar setting, using the same data collection instruments, would produce essentially the same results (see Blaxter *et al.* 1996: 200). However, some authors have gone so far as to question whether traditional concepts of validity, reliability and generalisability have any place at all within qualitative approaches (for example, Smith 1984; see Webb 1999: 324).

Absolute reliability would be impossible in a true action research study, as the individualistic, context-specific nature of the study should reflect its nuances and unique perspectives, most of which are the cultural product of the social interactions of those closely involved in bringing it about. When an action research study is judged, then, additional and more sensitive criteria have to be built in to see whether co-researchers have successfully engaged with each other in a genuine attempt at problem-solving.

The most important criterion for judging an action research study is whether it has *cultural validity*, that is, whether it provides a trustworthy and believable narrative of the problem under scrutiny. Would another practitioner in similar circumstances read it and recognise the problems or views expressed as similar to their own experiences? The usefulness of an action research study lies not only in resolving problems at the sharp end of practice, but also in generating debate on how others can do the same, albeit in different settings or areas of practice, and a project's success can be measured in how well it reaches out to other practitioners and offers them some tangible expression of hope in bringing about a better way of working together.

Validation techniques

Validation techniques which help to ground action research studies include:

- bringing in external observers or verifiers;
- replicating interventions in different settings;
- using methodological 'triangulation';
- duplicating the critical analysis of different data sets to see whether opinions agree or show consistent discrepancies; and
- peer review.

One way of increasing the accuracy of collected data is to use multiple observers of the same event who work independently and then compare written records (Barton-Cunningham 1993: 147). *Insider verifying* means that the data and its interpretation may be checked and re-checked with those carrying out the intervention. *Outsider verifying* by contrast means bringing in 'significant disinterested colleagues' to see whether they agree or disagree with the findings of different sets of data (*ibid.* 147).

Replication involves repeating the same data collection methods in either the same setting but using a different group of co-researchers, or in a similar setting which shares most of the characteristics of the first. When analysing data used in this way you try to identify the frequency with which similar positions or concepts and ideas occur, and whether any discrepancies identified are consistent across several settings. High levels of frequency and consistency together produce a 'valid' account of your findings.

Anomalies need to be accounted for, too, however, and should not be ignored. Data which does not fit should be accepted, reported and cherished, according to Blaxter and her colleagues: 'It is not uncommon for accepted interpretations to be challenged and eventually demolished. Do not cast aside pieces of data which may be the basis for doing this!' (Blaxter *et al.* 1996: 199).

Methodological triangulation involves using different data collection instruments and techniques to observe or glean information on the same phenomenon. Some researchers believe that triangulation can improve validity and overcome the biases inherent in a single perspective. *Theoretical triangulation* refers to the use of different theoretical perspectives in the study of a particular problem (for a discussion on both see Holloway 1997: 157).

Evidently, the more times the phenomenon or problem is investigated, the more perspectives that emerge. The skill of analysis in action research is in co-researchers working together to identify common themes and issues which have a direct relevance to the problem under investigation whatever the methods of data collection involved.

Above all, action research requires co-researchers to learn through personal and group relationships in what has been called the 'generative transformational order of communication' and the educative approach (Bohm 1983, see McNiff *et al.* 1992).

By *duplicating* the analysis of different sets of data, i.e. by asking co-researchers to analyse the data collected by other groups of co-researchers in the same study, it is also possible to identify commonalities and discrepancies. Sometimes this approach can lead to flashes of insight, or help to identify the 'psychic prisons' (Morgan 1986) which can encircle people, who are at times trapped within their own biases and uncritical modes of thinking. When does a belief become a prejudice, for example, or why are some explanations for a phenomenon given greater credence than others?

Challenging orthodoxies

Atkinson talks about the 'orthodoxies of medical thought' which saturate medical thinking and action. His research set out to 'examine how the facts of medically defined disease are produced and shared between medical practitioners and others; how they persuade one another of the facts of the case; equally, how they construct the case itself; how senior clinicians coach and instruct students and junior colleagues and so reproduce the orthodoxies of medical thought, knowledge and talk' (Atkinson 1995: 5).

Thus when analysing data in action research co-researchers need to identify the orthodoxies of thought within their own disciplines or fields of practice, and learn to distinguish between orthodoxies which perpetuate uncritical or unequal power relations between colleagues and colleagues, practitioners and patients, and so on. How has that orthodoxy come about and what implications does it have for the study's aims as a whole?

As a proponent of critical thinking in adults, Brookfield might view this kind of examination as an exercise in 'political learning', politics being 'a shorthand term for the processes by which decisions are made, wealth is distributed, services are regulated, justice is maintained, and minority interests are protected' (Brookfield 1987: 164). Analysing our data is in itself a political act, because 'political learning is evident whenever people notice, and begin to ponder, the discrepancies and inequities among groups in their societies....Asking awkward questions about the rightness of, and justification for, political decisions, actions, and structures is the focus of critical thinking in the political world' (*ibid.* 165).

Whether these questions apply to clinical practice, care decisions or care evaluation, they are highly legitimate questions which action research has the ability to examine. Such analysis is risky, however, as it asks people to dispense with their normal psychological defence mechanisms (lies, rationalisations, euphemisms and excuses!). In asking critical questions the researcher is engaging in refutation, entering into an exploratory dialogue with others about what is the right and the best course of action. As Seeskin would have it: this is only 'destructive in order to be therapeutic – like the doctor who must cut and burn in order to heal' (Seeskin 1987: 5).

Clearly, co-researchers who engage in this kind of analysis have a responsibility to be vigilant to the possibility that emotional damage or offence may be caused by their critical questioning and analysis. When probing and exploring values in the workplace, tact and sensitivity are required to ensure that researchers do not create problems on their own account.

Peer review is an integral part of the action research philosophy and is interwoven throughout. Collaborative analysis which allows individual co-researchers to constantly compare the findings of their data across different work and client settings helps to clarify problem areas and can encourage a group cohesiveness that may not have been strong beforehand. Additional peer review also takes place when the first draft of an action research report is circulated and of course at the stage of the final report when an account is published and disseminated further.

Self-validation also occurs when practitioners recognise the need to engage in critical reflection, in their 'desire to explore an intuitive understanding of practice and communicate it to others' (McNiff 1988: 132). *Learner validation* is often the outcome of dialogues between co-researchers in a study and can emerge from support group meetings where individuals compare their own feelings and findings and assess 'how far they have come' in their own appraisal of the subject being studied (*ibid.* 135).

Exploring your data

Analysis of data in action research therefore occurs at several levels.

(1) At the level of transcription and sorting of data.
(2) In the critical analysis of the content of the data by co-researchers.
(3) In the discussion over whether the data produced 'tells the story accurately, faithfully and intelligently'.
(4) In the formal evaluation of the action research process, i.e. perceived success in posing a solution to the problem identified and generating further insightful questions.

Overall, your data should provide you with the clues necessary to provide answers to the questions posed in Table 4.1.

By 'mapping' the answers to these questions from your data you should be able to develop your thinking and devise further data collecting instruments (if necessary) which are sensitive to the subtle cues presented by the existing data. As the problem is

Table 4.1 Exploring your data.

- What are the *key concepts* or issues running through the study? Have *central arguments* been identified? What is the problem being studied *attributed to*? Have any *barriers to effective practice* been identified?
- *How are these barriers constructed and by whom*, and have they been challenged or changed by co-researchers in any way? How can such a challenge be made effectively and *ethically*? Do other *agencies* need to consulted?
- Have *key players* been identified? Whose *logistical support* will need to be enlisted to help solve the problem? If *remedial action* is being resisted what are the reasons for this and whose interests are being protected or exposed by this?
- What *key assumptions* have co-researchers made about the problem? Can these be justified? What *beliefs* or *values* are expressed in the data and what impact do these have on resolving the problem? To be successful, will co-researchers require colleagues and others outside of the study to join them in a 'culture shift' of these beliefs and *adaptation* to a new position? What *feelings* has the study generated? How have *emotions* been expressed and how have they helped (or delayed) the problem-solving process?

---

unpicked, a stitch at a time in much the same way as a piece of embroidery or a tapestry might be, it becomes possible to see where problematic knots and tangles in the weave of practice lie. The situation then needs to be reworked, bringing together the new image or vision generated by co-researchers in the field.

The time to stop collecting data is when you feel you have reached saturation point in your analysis, that is, when it seems that you have enough evidence to support emerging key findings and you are satisfied that you will be able to create 'a recognizable reality' for readers in your report of the process (see Maykut & Morehouse 1994: 126).

Some researchers use additional field notes to guide their analysis, an example of which can be found in McKernan (1991). Others rely on a personal diary of events which carefully documents different stages and tasks in the research process, where they might include personal thoughts and ideas relating to their analysis of the data. All these may be legitimately included as data in their own right, although individuals do have a right of privacy as regards their use and may therefore prefer to keep these for personal reference only.

Having collected and analysed the data, the next stage is to ascertain whether your actions and discoveries have moved the problem forward. *Evaluative questions* now need to be asked so that your final report not only describes your research but also the implications of key findings for future practice and care.

Evaluative questions

These questions relate to the overall outcome of the research process and give you a basis on which to construct your draft of findings. Looking critically at all the data that has been analysed and all the things that have happened over the research period, write down the answers to the following questions.

Has any progress been made in resolving the initial research question or problem? Describe this in no more than twelve sentences.

Are co-researchers confident that findings are a faithful representation of practice? Describe the overall position in no more than ten sentences.

Do the findings challenge or add to established theory in this area? Justify this in no more than twenty sentences.

Has any new theory or concept emerged from your study and, if so, how may this be retested and re-evaluated by colleagues in your particular discipline or field of practice? Explain the situation in no more than twenty sentences.

Who stands to be affected by the findings of your study and does this raise any ethical dilemmas prior to publishing the results? Ask this question very carefully by considering all the stakeholders and their respective positions both before and after your study. Summarise your conclusions in no more than twenty sentences.

Why did you choose action research and how was it managed in relation to (a) data collection, (b) data analysis, (c) ethical practice? Account for your practice in no more than thirty sentences.

What you have written should provide you with the central arguments for your draft report. In order to abide by the collaborative nature of the study, you may ask other co-researchers to complete the same exercise independently and then come together to discuss the result. This acts as an additional safeguard in making sure that your study accurately reflects events, and also helps to clarify sticking points or any areas of uncertainty.

If your study is small-scale this may not be open to you, in which case you should share your report with your supervisor(s) and your mentor if they are interested. Mentors can be very good at spotting your prejudices as they probably know you and your approach to work very well. Limit the number of readers as too many opinions may leave you sidetracked and confused.

Drafting your report

There are different ways of providing an account of your study and you may have to produce several accounts in order to satisfy different audiences. An academic thesis (and the accompanying viva examination) will be judged on different criteria than the kind of reports that sponsors or employers will find useful.

For comprehensive and constructive advice on thesis preparation and submission and on surviving the viva see Holloway & Walker (1999) which details the process from the perspective of research students in health and social care.

Most sponsors and employers will appreciate both an *executive summary of findings* and a more detailed account in a *full report*. In many ways it is the former which will be most read by policy-makers, while policy-drivers (those responsible for implementing policy at local level) will be interested in the rationale behind your recommendations, and will want to see whether their own situations have much in common with the settings you have described. In general, both pieces of work will need to be comprehensible to your readers, presented in language which is clear and easy to understand and which is not drowned in jargon or complex analyses of issues which are of only peripheral interest.

Funding agencies generally want to know that their money has been well spent and like to see tangible results for their patronage. It is important therefore to identify clearly key issues which can be reported back to all agencies involved with the minimum of fuss. Attention to detail is important, but if you are being pressured into publishing earlier than you had hoped (or if you are running considerably behind your original time schedule) it is better to communicate your key findings, indicating that a more detailed account is being polished for subsequent peer review and dissemination. Given that action research is a cyclical process, it is possible to put one foot to the ground occasionally before pedalling your way to the finish.

One of the main issues which trouble action researchers (and lead researchers in particular) is when to withdraw from the setting and to call your study complete. If the intervention has been successful it may come to a natural conclusion, with no further lead researcher involvement being required. The ethos of action research should remain, however, in that practitioners now have the means to go on and research further issues in practice for themselves. Only you can tell when you have reached the stage of saturation, when there is little more of value that you can do or oversee on behalf of co-researchers, or when you sense that co-researcher fatigue is setting in.

An executive summary should be no more than two A4 sides of single spaced type. A full report may contain up to 15 000 words. Some sponsors specify length and format in advance and it is wise to follow these closely.

The length of an academic dissertation or thesis is, of course, more substantial as you are required to provide a comprehensive justification of all the elements of your study. Guidance on this should be available from your academic supervisor, and your university will provide a copy of the relevant degree regulations to you on request.

It is important not to leave this too late, however, as you do not want any surprises at the writing up stage. Read the small print of the regulations and this will give you an indication of how your work is to be set out, how illustrations and tables should be presented and, critically, the deadlines you must observe for your work to be considered.

Extensions to the study period can sometimes be negotiated, but only if you have a very good reason (ill-health or a family bereavement, for example). Not all universities are equally sympathetic or work to the same guidelines, so it is worth consulting your supervisor as soon as you have any indication at all that your work may be affected.

Issues in writing up collaboratively

Some people avoid action research because of concerns about the collaborative nature of writing up. They worry that 'too many cooks may spoil the broth' and that there will be disagreements over what should be included in the final work. The ability of participants to adhere to deadlines may vary and bad feeling can result if one party feels let down by another who promised to contribute something but then failed to do so. The lead researcher has the overall responsibility for writing up as he or she will usually have initiated the study in the first place. It would seem only practical and fair, however, to expect other co-researchers to contribute by writing up a particular aspect of the study. Realistically, few co-researchers are in a position to do more than take responsibility for one or two sections of your report. The dissertation and thesis may take account of these contributions (and indeed must acknowledge them fully), but the writing up of your academic work should be yours alone.

Some action researchers get round the writing problem by sharing out aspects of writing based on preferences expressed by co-researchers. This can often be tied to opportunities for co-publication at a later stage, when colleagues can draft articles together for submission to the professional journals. This provides an added incentive and gives added value to participation, particularly if this can then be included in the practitioner's portfolio and used to demonstrate professional development to employers. Co-publication is sometimes the first opportunity a professional has to venture into the world of publishing, and the opportunity to collaborate in all the processes of production as a group can be an exciting and unanticipated departure for some practitioners, particularly if they have not been part of a research culture to date.

Once you have completed your draft report this should be made available to co-researchers who then read it and supply clarification or comments. References should be accurate to avoid any misunderstandings about the sources of material. When you have all agreed on the draft, a final report can be set out which covers:

- details of the research problem or question;
- an explanation of the action research process and a justification of your methods of data collection;
- an overview of the literature review process and the implications of your study in relation to established thinking or practice;
- an indication of your key findings and their implications for practice;
- an indication of questions or issues raised by the study for future reference;
- a summary of how you intend to disseminate your work and build on it for the future; and
- acknowledgement of all those involved in, or who supported, your study.

Battista *et al.* (1994) point out that the communication of pertinent information can have an important effect on the shaping of our health care systems. Policy makers 'interpret research in a context of societal priorities; they are vulnerable to the biases of individual scientists and experts, and their environment predisposes them to accept scientific information that is politically convenient' (Battista *et al.* 1994: 25).

Qualitative studies in particular can face problems in being taken seriously for practice, as they may be seen as too 'soft' or unreliable for general use. Much can be overcome by careful presentation of your final report, however, as Jones (1994) advises. When asked to present your report remember first of all to engage your audience. 'Pose a vital question using arresting visual or written material and communicate your own enthusiasm for the subject'. Describe the context of your report so that it is crystal clear, make connections with previous published work and help them to see why your work is so relevant. Emphasise the novelty of your findings. Avoid tedious or repetitive formats. Take time to explain what you have achieved in ways that stimulate interest and have people making connections to their own practice and areas of responsibility (Jones 1994: 53).

Above all, make yourself available to discuss the results and to bring others on board in the interests of dissemination and practitioner development. Be prepared to see the study from the perspective of other professionals or client groups. Occasionally studies have been known to generate new projects in other areas and so the research community widens and service users benefit as a result of new ideas and new-found enthusiasm. Be prepared to speak publicly about your achievements and to take advice on presentation and public speaking if you need to. Support your co-researchers in conducting their own local dissemination and perhaps by preparing a concurrent session or poster presentation for the benefit of interested groups and professional societies. Submit your findings to relevant journals (taking care to read their guidelines first), and do not feel dejected if your work is returned. Editors will usually offer constructive advice on your paper; alternatively your academic supervisor may have suggestions as to how you can develop your work.

Morse (1994: 59) has some excellent advice on writing up, and as an experienced and authoritative writer on qualitative health research, her advice can save many hours of worry. Jones advises that the deadliest enemy of any researcher is isolation, something with which many researchers identify (Jones 1994). Action research should provide a reasonable defence against loneliness in researchers, but it is often in the writing process that doubts begin to creep in and that a personal sense of confidence waivers. Just how do you reduce weeks and months (sometimes years) of work, discussion and argument into so few words?

Remember, in action research what you write is only a small part of the process. What really matters is that you brought practitioners together to discuss an issue of social relevance and importance; you enabled them to work together and to think critically about their situations. Those skills and attributes developed through involvement with your study will stay with them as they develop their careers.

Action research can and does change the world (if only in one place at a time), and you can be assured that unlike other less 'active' research, the impact of your study will be felt in some form, somewhere, long after the dust has finally settled on any written report.

APPENDIX

Guidelines for critiquing action research

The value of a research paper depends on three main issues according to Avis (1994b). These are the relevance of the research objectives, the validity of the evidence, and the sufficiency of the evidence provided to support claims made in the authors' conclusion (Avis 1994b: 276).

When it comes to critiquing action research we can safely add many other criteria and these are set out below. You may decide to use them as a checklist for you own research prior to final submission, or as a tool to measure the success of your study or project at different stages in the research process. They are intended to be used flexibly and to focus your attention on the central issues. An alternative is to divide them up into sections and to give co-researchers responsibility for overseeing one or two of them as the research progresses. This helps to keep you on track and enables you to see where potential weaknesses in your study may lie. If you are planning or undertaking your own study as a lead researcher, you can refer back to this list from time to time for your own peace of mind and use the list as a kind of quality assurance mechanism or indicator.

The questions are not set in stone, but are an idea of the kinds of questions experienced researchers may want to ask. They have been divided into categories, some of which may have more or less relevance to you depending on the style and substance of your work. The categories are:

- Research aims
- Study management
- Learning outcomes
- Outcomes for policy and practice
- Quality of report
- Validity
- Value Added, i.e. the extra bonuses accrued from participation which should be communicated to co-researchers, sponsors and employers.

Additional questions may be added to reflect the particular ethos and flavour of your own study.

Research aims

Have the researchers been clear about their research intentions? _____

Is the research question or problem clear and unambiguous? _____

Has the initiative been sustained over time? _____

Is it possible to see how one development led to another? _____

Have problem-solving processes been made explicit? _____

How well do the outcomes compare to the stated aims of the
research as outlined at the beginning? _____

Study management

Have sufficient steps been taken to ensure that everyone who needs
to be informed has been kept informed? _____

Was formal permission for access sought and was written consent
obtained for the study? _____

Have any threats to the study's survival been dealt with in an ethical
and constructive manner? _____

Have the rights of co-researchers, colleagues, clients and patients
been communicated and protected? _____

Have unexpected problems been managed effectively? _____

Have ethical issues been thought through, anticipated and dealt with
in a professional way? _____

Is there sound evidence of co-researcher input, e.g. have feedback
processes worked well? _____

Learning outcomes

What have co-researchers learned from the experience?

Is the intended culture or policy change evident in the findings?

Have any outcomes completely surprised co-researchers?

How have co-researchers developed as a group or team?

What new skills or attributes have been acquired through participation and what implications does this have for the group and individuals?

Has the experience been a positive one and if not, why? What could future researchers learn from this?

Outcomes for policy and practice

What changes and/or improvements have been made to policy and practice as a result of this study?

Is there evidence to suggest that improvements will be maintained?

Have stakeholders and potential stakeholders been informed of these outcomes and their relevance?

Have sponsors been kept informed of progress and have their priorities been borne in mind by the study and the final report?

Have any new questions or issues emerged as a result of the study? If so, are the implications of these recognised and summarised?

Quality of report

Is the report clear and the narrative continuous?

Is the analysis thorough and consistent?

Does the analysis reflect and respect diversity of opinion?

Is the report well presented, accurately referenced and interesting to read?

Is the literature review authoritative and inclusive of key concepts? Is collaboration evident?

Validity

Has the study's setting been an appropriate and relevant one for the question or problem identified? _____

Are the experiences and opinions of participants well described? _____

Do the feelings and outcomes of the study read as a genuine and authentic attempt to uncover the explanations and understandings of others? _____

Is the study believable? Does it make sense to you as an experienced practitioner? _____

Has the study been genuinely collaborative? _____

Value added

Have co-researchers enjoyed and benefited from the experience? _____

Is there evidence of increased group cohesiveness and better team working? _____

Have the problem-solving abilities of co-researchers improved? _____

Have any residual problems or bonuses been identified? _____

Have attitudes towards research-based practice changed at all as a result of involvement? _____

Have any 'loose ends' emerged which need to be addressed or tidied up in the interests of researcher professionalism? _____

Is there evidence that interest in the subject being studied will continue after the report has been published? _____

Is there evidence of planned dissemination involving all co-researchers and not just the lead researcher? _____

Would your reading of and/or involvement in this study encourage further participation in action research? If the answer to this question is no, it would be helpful to elaborate on why and to see whether you need to expand on the strengths and limitations in an article or paper of your own for the benefit of other researchers and practitioners.

References

Adair, J. (1988) *Effective Time Management: how to save time and spend it wisely.* Pan Books, London.

Adams, J., Hayes, J., Hopson, B. (1976) *Transition: understanding and managing personal change.* Martin Robertson, London.

Alasuutari, P. (1998) *An Invitation to Social Research.* Sage, London.

Appleyard, B. (1999) *Brave New Worlds: genetics and the human experience.* Harper Collins, London.

Atkinson, P. (1995) *Medical Talk and Medical Work: the liturgy of the clinic.* Sage, London.

Avis, M. (1994a) Reading research critically. I. An introduction to appraisal: designs and objectives. *Journal of Clinical Nursing*, **3**, 227–234.

Avis, M. (1994b) Reading Research Critically. II. An introduction to appraisal: assessing the evidence, *Journal of Clinical Nursing*, **3**, 271–277.

Bamford, M., Wilkes, J., Pope, A., Edwards, A., Jordan, K., Warder, J. (1998) *Nurse Led Minor Injuries Services: an evaluative study into nursing interventions.* Centre for Health Planning and Management, University of Keele.

Barton-Cunningham, J. (1993) *Action Research and Organisational Development.* Praeger Publishers, Westport, Connecticut.

Battista, R.N., Ruiz, E.A., Endicott, A.N. (1994) From Science to Practice: the evolving art of communication. In: *Disseminating Research/Changing Practice* (eds E.V. Dunn, P.G. Norton, M. Stewart, F. Tudiver, M.J. Bass), pp. 21–31. Research Methods for Primary Care, Vol. 6. Sage, Thousand Oaks, California.

Beck, U. (1992) *Risk Society: towards a new modernity.* Sage, London.

Berkman, L. F. (1984) Assessing the Physical Health Effects of Social Networks and Social Support. *Annual Review of Public Health*, **5**, 413–432.

Blaxter, L., Hughes, C., Tight, M. (1996) *How to Research.* Open University Press, Buckingham.

Bohm, D. (1983) *Wholeness and the Implicate Order*. Ark Paperbacks, London.

Breda, K. (1997) Enhanced Nursing Autonomy through Participatory Action Research. *Nursing Outlook*, March/April, **45**(2), 76–81.

Bridges, W. (1996) *Making Sense of Life's Changes*. Nicholas Brealey, London.

Brookfield, S.D. (1987) *Developing Critical Thinkers: challenging adults to new ways of thinking and acting*. Open University Press, Milton Keynes.

Broome, A.K. (1990) *Managing Change*. Macmillan, Basingstoke.

Burrows, D. (1997) Action on Pain. In: *Nurse Teachers as Researchers: a reflective approach* (ed. S. Thompson). Edward Arnold, London.

Cohen S. & Wills, T.A. (1985) Stress, Social Support and the Buffering Hypothesis. *Psychological Bulletin*, **98**, 310–357.

Crompton, R., Gallie, D., Purcell, K. (1996) *Changing Forms of Employment: organisations, skills and gender*. Routledge, London.

Dallos, R. (1996) Creating Relationships: patterns of actions and beliefs. In: *Social Interaction and Personal Relationships* (eds D. Meisl & R. Dallos). Sage/Open University, Milton Keynes.

Dey, I. (1993) *Qualitative Data Analysis: a user-friendly guide for social scientists*. Routledge, London.

Doyle, R. (1996) Breaking the Solitudes to Improve Services for Ethnic Groups: action research strategies. In: *The Reflective Researcher: social workers' theories of practice research* (ed. J. Fook). Allen & Unwin, St Leonards, Australia.

Easterby-Smith, M., Thorpe, R., Lowe, A. (1991) *Management Research: an introduction*. Sage, London.

Elliott, J. (1991) *Action Research for Educational Change*. Open University Press, Buckingham.

Fisher, S. (1990) *On the Move: the psychological effects of change and transition*. Chichester: John Wiley.

Fiske, M. & Chiriboga, D.A. (1990) *Change and Continuity in Adult Life*. Jossey-Bass, San Francisco.

Freire, P. (1972) *Pedagogy of the Oppressed*. Herder & Herder, New York.

Gibson, C.H. (1991) A Concept Analysis of Empowerment. *Journal of Advanced Nursing*, **16**, 354–361.

Harper, M. & Hartman, N. (1997) Research Paradigms. In: *Research-Mindedness for Practice: an interactive approach for nursing and health care* (ed. P. Smith), pp. 20–52. Churchill Livingstone, Edinburgh.

Hart, E. & Bond, M. (1995) *Action Research for Health and Social Care: a guide to practice*. Open University Press, Buckingham.

Holloway, I. (1997) *Basic Concepts for Qualitative Research*. Blackwell Science, Oxford.

Holloway, I. & Walker, S. (1999) *Getting a PhD in Health and Social Care*. Blackwell Science, Oxford.

Holloway, I. & Wheeler, S. (1996) *Qualitative Research for Nurses*. Blackwell Science, Oxford.

Holter, I.M. & Schwartz-Barcott, D. (1993) Action Research: What is it? How has it been used and how can it be used in nursing? *Journal of Advanced Nursing*, **18**, 289–304.

Hope, K. (1998) Starting Out with Action Research. *Nurse Researcher*, **6**(2), 16–26.

Jennings, L.E. (1995) Prisoners of Our Own Perspectives: recasting action research in modern/postmodern times. *Studies in Continuing Education*, **17**(1&2), 78–85.

Jones, R. (1994) Disseminating New Knowledge to Other Researchers. In: *Disseminating Research/Changing Practice* (eds E.V. Dunn, P.G. Norton, M. Stewart, F. Tudiver, M.J. Bass) pp. 45–58. Sage, Thousand Oaks, California.

Lantos, J.D. (1997) *Do We Still Need Doctors?* Routledge, New York & London.

Lathlean, J. (1997) Ethical Dimensions of Action Research. In: *Nursing Research: an ethical and legal appraisal* (ed. L. de Raeve), pp. 32–41. Bailliere Tindall, London.

Layder, D. (1993) *New Strategies in Social Research: an introduction and guide.* Polity Press, Cambridge.

Lewin, K. (1948) The Group Decision and Social Change. In: *Readings in Social Psychology* (ed. E. Maccoby). Holt, Rhinehart & Winston, London.

Marrow, C. (1998) Keeping Above the Surface in an Action Research Study. *Nurse Researcher*, **6**(2), 57–70.

Mason, D.J., Costello-Nickitas, D., Scanlan, J.M., Magnuson, B.A. (1991) Empowering Nurses for Politically Astute Change in the Workplace. *Journal of Continuing Education in Nursing*, **22**(1), 5–10.

Mason, J. (1996) *Qualitative Researching*. Sage, London.

Maykut, P. Morehouse, R. (1994) *Beginning Qualitative Research: a philosophic and practical guide*. Falmer Press, London.

Maynard, M. Purvis, J. (1994) *Researching Women's Lives from a Feminist Perspective*. Taylor & Francis, London.

McKernan, J. (1991) *Curriculum Action Research: a handbook of methods and resources for the reflective practitioner*. Kogan Page, London.

McNiff, J. (1988) *Action Research: principles and practice*. Routledge, London.

McNiff, J. Whitehead, J. Laidlaw, M. & members of the Bath Action Research Group (1992) *Creating a Good Social Order through Action Research*. Hyde Publications, Dorset.

Merriam, S.B. & Yang, B. (1996) A Longitudinal Study of Adult Life Experiences and Developmental Outcomes. *Adult Education Quarterly*, **46**(2), Winter, 62–81.

Morgan, G. (1986) *Images of Organization*. Sage, London.

Morse, J.M. (1994) Disseminating Qualitative Research. In: *Disseminating*

Research/Changing Practice (eds E.V. Dunn, P.G. Norton, M. Stewart, F. Tudiver, M.J. Bass) pp. 59–75. Sage, Thousand Oaks, California.

Moyer, A., Coristine, M., Jamault, M., Roberge, G., O'Hagan, M. (1999) Identifying Older People in Need Using Action Research. *Journal of Clinical Nursing,* **8**, 103–111.

Neumann, J.E., Kellner, K., Dawson-Shepherd, A. (1997) *Developing Organisational Consultancy*. Routledge, London.

Nichols, R., Meyer, J., Batehup, L., Waterman, H. (1997) Promoting Action Research in Health Care Settings. *Nursing Standard,* **11**(40), 36–38.

Nolan, M. & Grant, G. (1993) Action Research and Quality of Care: a mechanism for agreeing basic values as a precursor to change. *Journal of Advanced Nursing,* **18**, 305–311.

Pietroni, P. (1998). Foreword. In: *Critical Reading for the Reflective Practitioner* (eds R. Clarke & P. Croft). Butterworth-Heinemann, Oxford.

Powell, J. & Lovelock R. (1991) Negotiating with Agencies. In: *Handbook for Research Students in the Social Sciences* (eds G. Allan & C. Skinner), pp. 128–139. Falmer Press, London.

Radley, A. (1994) *Making Sense of Illness: the social psychology of health and disease*. Sage, London.

Ragin, C.C. (1994) *Constructing Social Research: the unity and diversity of method*. Sage, Thousand Oaks, California.

Robson, C. (1993) *Real World Research: a resource for social scientists and practitioner-researchers*. Blackwell Publishers, Oxford.

Rolfe, G. (1996) Going to Extremes: action research, grounded practice and the theory-practice gap in nursing. *Journal of Advanced Nursing,* **24**, 1315–1320.

Rolfe, G. (1998a) The Theory Practice Gap in Nursing: from research-based practice to practitioner-based research. *Journal of Advanced Nursing,* **28**(3), 672–679.

Rolfe, G. (1998b) *Expanding Nursing Knowledge: understanding and researching your own practice*. Butterworth-Heinemann, Oxford.

Rolfe, G. & Phillips, L. (1997) The Development and Evaluation of the Role of an Advanced Nurse Practitioner in Dementia: an action research project. *International Journal of Nursing Studies,* **34**(2), 119–127.

Schneider, S.C. & Barsoux, J.L. (1997) *Managing Across Cultures*. Prentice Hall, London.

Schon, D. (1971) *Beyond the Stable State*. Temple Smith, London.

Schratz, M. & Walker, R. (1995) *Research as Social Change: new opportunities for qualitative research*. Routledge, London.

Seeskin, K. (1987) *Dialogue and Discovery: a study in Socratic method*. SUNY Press, New York.

Shakespeare, P. (1993) Performing. In: *Reflecting on Research Practice: issues in health and social welfare* (eds P. Shakespeare, D. Atkinson, S. French), pp. 95–105. Open University Press, Buckingham.

Smart, B. (1996) Postmodern Social Theory. In: *The Blackwell Companion to Social Theory* (ed. B.S. Turner), pp. 396–428. Blackwell Publishers, Oxford.

Smith, J.K. (1984) The Problem of Criteria for Judging Interpretive Research. *Educational Evaluation and Policy Analysis*, **6**, 379–391.

Smith, P. (1997) *Research-Mindedness for Practice: an interactive approach for nursing and health care*. Churchill Livingstone, Edinburgh.

Stead, V. & Lee, M. (1996) Intercultural Perspectives on HRD. In: *Human Resource Development: perspectives, strategies and practice* (ed. J. Stewart, J. McGoldrick.), pp. 47–70. Pitman Publishing, London.

Stringer, P. (1996) *Action Research: a handbook for practitioners*. Avebury Press, Aldershot.

Tesch, R. (1990) *Qualitative Research: analysis types and software tools*. Falmer Press, London and Philadelphia.

Tierney, A. (1997) Planning and Managing an Action Research Project to Time. *Nurse Researcher*, **5**(1), 35–50.

Turner, B.S. (1995) *Medical Power and Social Knowledge*. Sage, London.

Underwood, F. & Parker, J. (1998) Developing and Evaluating an Acute Stroke Pathway through Action Research. *Nurse Researcher*, **6**(2), 27–38.

Wallis, S. (1998) Changing Practice Through Action Research. *Nurse Researcher*, 6(2), 5–15.

Webb, C. (1999) Analysing Qualitative Data: computerized and other approaches. *Journal of Advanced Nursing*, **29**(2), 323–330.

Weil, S. (1997) Postgraduate Education and Lifelong Learning as Collaborative Inquiry in Action: an emergent model. In: *Beyond the First Degree* (ed. R. Burgess), pp. 119–139. SRHE/Open University, Buckingham.

Weil, S. (1998) From Dearing and Systemic Control to Post Dearing and Systemic Inquiry: re-creating universities for 'Beyond the Stable State'. *Conference paper*.

Whyte, W.F. (1991) *Participatory Action Research*, Focus edn. Sage, Newbury Park, California.

Wilkinson, R.G. (1996) *Unhealthy Societies: the afflictions of inequality*. Routledge, London.

Williams, P.L. & Webb, C. (1994) The Delphi Technique: a methodological discussion. *Journal of Advanced Nursing*, **19**, 180–186.

Winter, R. (1989) *Learning from Experience: Principles and Practice in Action Research*. Falmer Press, London.

Winter, R. (1996) Some Principles and Procedures for the Conduct of Action Research. In: *New Directions in Action Research* (ed. O. Zuber-Skerritt), pp. 13–27. Falmer Press, London.

Zuber-Skerritt, O. (1996) *New Directions in Action Research*. Falmer Press, London.

Further reading

The range of texts on research methods and on the philosophy of social research is vast. The recommendations which follow are a personal choice and most are included with the needs of the beginning researcher or practitioner-researcher in mind.

Allan, G. & Skinner, C. (1991) *Handbook for Research Students in the Social Sciences*. Falmer Press, London.

Blaxter, L., Hughes, C., Tight, M. (1996) *How to Research*. Open University Press, Buckingham.

Cassell, C. & Symon, G. (1994*) Qualitative Methods in Organizational Research: a practical guide*. Sage, London.

Cerinus, M. (1999) What Price Research? Good Preparation Contributes to Good Performance. *Nursing Standard,* 13(49), 32–37.

Dane, F.C. (1990) *Research Methods*. Brooks Cole, Pacific Grove, California.

Edwards, A. & Talbot, R. (1994) *The Hard-Pressed Researcher: a research handbook for the caring professions.* Longman, Harlow.

Hart, E. & Bond, M. (1995) *Action Research for Health and Social Care*. Open University Press, Buckingham,

Holloway, I. (1997) *Basic Concepts for Qualitative Research*. Blackwell Science, Oxford.

Holloway, I. & Wheeler, S. (1996) *Qualitative Research for Nurses*. Blackwell Science, Oxford.

Kleinman S. & Copp, M.A. (1993) *Emotions and Fieldwork*. Sage, Newbury Park, California.

Lee, R.M. (1993) *Doing Research on Sensitive Topics*. Sage, London.

Mason, J. (1996) *Qualitative Researching*. Sage, London.

Reason, P. (1994) *Participation in Human Inquiry*. Sage, London.

Robinson, V. (1993) *Problem-Based Methodology: research for the improvement of practice*. Oxford, Pergamon.

Sapsford, R. & Abbott, P. (1992) *Research Methods for Nurses and the Caring Professions*. Open University Press, Buckingham.

Warren, C.A.B. (1988) *Gender Issues in Field Research*. Sage, Newbury Park, California.

For background in change theory

Broome, A.K. (1990) *Managing Change*. Macmillan, London

Carnall, C.(1995) *Managing Change in Organisations*. Prentice Hall, London.

Index